DATE DUE

GOD'S COUNTRY:
A CASE AGAINST THEOCRACY
Sandy Rapp

SOME ADVANCE REVIEWS

God's Country is a much needed primer on the premises of personal privacy underlying lesbian/gay civil rights and reproductive freedom. All personal liberties are dramatically threatened by the contemporary religious right's unending crusade to legislate sectarian beliefs. To read this book is to view these "social issues" from psychological, political, and religious perspectives. *God's Country* is a must for Americans interested in preserving their country's historic commitment to freedom for the individual.

The Honorable Bella Abzug
Former Congresswoman from New York

The way of dictatorship everywhere begins by enlisting the self-righteous and God-fearing to abolish the moral evils of democratic sexual rights. Dictatorship then encroaches upon all the democratic rights of free citizens as moral evils and abolishes them. Americans today are already imperiled by an excessively dangerous amount of religious dictatorship in government. Read Sandy Rapp's book and awake to the peril.

John Money, PhD
Director, Psychohormonal Research Unit
Professor of Medical Psychology and
Professor of Pediatrics, Emeritus
The Johns Hopkins Hospital and School of Medicine

God's Country
A Case Against Theocracy

HAWORTH Women's Studies
Ellen Cole and Esther Rothblum
Senior Co-Editors

New, Recent, and Forthcoming Titles

When Husbands Come Out of the Closet by Jean Schaar Gochros

Prisoners of Ritual: An Odyssey into Female Circumcision in Africa by Hanny Lightfoot-Klein

Foundations for a Feminist Restructuring of the Academic Disciplines edited by Michele Paludi and Gertrude A. Steuernagel

Hippocrates' Handmaidens: Women Married to Physicians by Esther Nitzberg

Waiting: A Diary of Loss and Hope in Pregnancy by Ellen Judith Reich

God's Country: A Case Against Theocracy by Sandy Rapp

Women and Aging: Celebrating Ourselves by Ruth Raymond Thone

A Woman's Odyssey into Africa: Tracks Across a Life by Hanny Lightfoot-Klein

Women's Conflicts About Eating and Sexuality: The Relationship Between Food and Sex by Rosalyn M. Meadow and Lillie Weiss

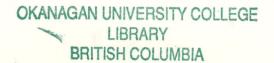
God's Country
A Case Against Theocracy

Sandy Rapp

The Haworth Press
New York • London • Sydney

The Haworth Press, Inc., 10 Alice Street, Binghamton, NY 13904-1580
EUROSPAN/Haworth, 3 Henrietta Street, London WC2E 8LU England
ASTAM/Haworth, 162-168 Parramatta Road, Stanmore (Sydney), N.S.W. 2048 Australia

Library of Congress Cataloging-in-Publication Data

Rapp, Sandy.
    God's country : a case against theocracy / Sandy Rapp.
      p. cm.
    Includes bibliographical references.
    Includes index.
    ISBN 1-56024-103-9 (alk. paper)
    1. United States—Social policy—1980- 2. Sociology, Christian—United States. 3. Religion and state—United States. 4. Sex and law—United States. 5. Homophobia—United States. 6. Sexism—United States. I. Title.
HN65.R37   1991
306.7'0973—dc20
                                                                        91-7771
                                                                             CIP

Thank you to

Anne L. Butler
for a lifetime of friendship and literary assistance

Deborah Ann Light
for office use and various philanthropies

John Jermain Library Staff
Sag Harbor, NY

with special thanks to

THE LINDA LEIBMAN HUMAN RIGHTS FUND
Bridgehampton, NY

CONTENTS

INTRODUCTION

In the past decade privacy rights and their underlying premises have sustained direct and incessant assault by a powerful, tax-exempt minority, energized with a fundamentalist religious zeal and such thoughts as "The idea of religion and politics don't mix was invented by the devil to keep Christians from running their own country" (frequent '80s White House guest Reverend Jerry Falwell in 1976).

This assault represents, more succinctly than any other crusade in history, a crystallization of the 2,500-year-old patriarchal agenda which has left this country such legacies as witch burnings, coat hanger abortions, and at least one minority exquisitely groomed as host to a sexually transmitted pandemic.

It is the thesis of this book that many U.S. citizens, numbers of whom represent profoundly affected categories (i.e., women—lesbian or non-gay, and gay men) do not understand what is happening, do not know how to counter what is happening, either do not know of or do not relate to existing strategies, and do not know how to apply such strategies as they have absorbed to situations in their immediate province.

God's Country: A Case Against Theocracy traces the patriarchal premises which underlie the 20th century crusade. While many works examine the sexist issues minutely, through the lenses of various focused fields, this book considers the whole elephant as opposed to a trunk, a tail, and a side. The idea is to unify the lesbian/gay—male/feminist arena with an interdisciplinary overview of sexual politics in historical, psychological, and religious perspectives. An attempt is also made to connect local educational efforts with national policies for people who wish the government out of their bedrooms but are not sure how it got there in the first place. It is this author's experience that many such persons lack the time to pursue those various philosophic and activist tracts that might deal with these matters vis-à-vis respective fields.

Particular attention is given to the fulcrum issues currently defended as "privacy rights" in their Constitutional presumption or lack thereof. Now daily front page fare, these issues range from gays in the military to the unavailability of safe, effective contraception in the United States.

But truly important advances have been made in the fields of psychology and religion, and such developments can be brought to bear upon the many doctrines and superstitions which are today being presented as scientific "facts." Chapters 1 through 3 deal with these psychological materials and their importance as a foundation for gay/lesbian civil rights. An attempt is also made to acquaint readers with the enormous psychological damage that is caused by erroneous information.

A short background of feminist thought is included and lesbian experience is considered specifically against the ground of larger misogyny. Although some readers will be familiar with the background material, I am convinced that there also exists a growing body of alarmed rights-conscious citizens who might welcome a review of this old feminist territory.

Chapter 4 recreates a particularly hairy legislative hearing, replete with anti-gay fundamentalist Christians. Chapter 5 addresses abortion as a pivotal issue in sexual politics. A history is drawn up with an eye on the current Catholic perspective and the relatively recent adoption thereof. The 1989 Webster decision is used as a lens upon various Constitutional outlooks, and theological pro-choice positions are discussed. Also considered is the ongoing U.S. exportation of pronatalism abroad.

Chapter 6 submits that the Bible is not a history of God's word, but rather a collection of mythologies and teachings, some of which date far beyond the Judeo/Christian father-god to early Pagan times of matrifocal and gender-balanced theologies. (The adjective "Pagan" is capitalized to offset the religion's persistent subsumption as a primitive backdrop against which patriarchy's majesty emerged.) Contemporary scholars explain that much misinterpretation has befallen scripture in its countless translations. And it is shown that passages which now seem to impugn lesbians and gay men had no such meaning in the original texts. Such developments show that the zealots' biblical interpretation is not universal moral precept, but rather a specific sectarian view which adherents have every right to hold but no right whatever to impose across the board in the United States.

The work ends with the beginnings of patriarchal dissolution in the New Age. Some contemporary "channeled" writings on the privacy issues are included in Chapter 7. Of course the spiritual "revelations" of the present are no more or less amenable to proof than are those of the past. But such perspectives are broadening and provide an even wider philosophic standing from which to consider the subjects. I close with a short "how to" chapter about available national resources. Some language and positions which have proved effective in various legislative and educational efforts are reviewed and a few usable examples of letters to the editor are provided.

As a lesbian and a woman's rights activist, I also have certain personal perspectives which are incorporated throughout the presentation. My habit is to formally relate the information and then interpret it somewhat colloquially. I have found the mix works well with most audiences, and I hope the occasional splashes of grassroots color do not offend serious readers.

REFERENCE KEY

Most reference notes for this book are contained in the text itself. Paragraphs with quotes and citings also include names (and dates when authors have multiple cites) through which readers may locate sources in the Bibliography. Occasional bracketed name and date references also refer readers to the Bibliography. The Bibliography itself contains information about chapters and pages of cited works.

CHAPTER 1

A GAY MALE EXPERIENCE

"Cocksuckers," demurred Yale Biology Professor Alvin Novick, MD, to an AIDS and Civil Liberties forum in Bridgehampton, New York on August 21, 1987. He took in a scattering of thin lips, tightened as the more conservative audience members reacted to the word. "Cocksuckers," he repeated, and expressly identified himself as a gay male. "It's your word — not mine, you know," he added to emphasize that such terms did not originate in the lesbian/gay community. Dr. Novick went on to lambaste the heterosexist orthodoxy imposed upon impressionable young people who are encouraged, nay required, to despise sissies: "We are all enrolled in a course one might call Bigotry 101, so that when some of us first experience longings for other men and boys we think that it can't be so because we know we are not those despicable sissies, fags, and cocksuckers we've been beating up for years . . ."

By no stretch of the imagination does Dr. Novick exaggerate society's stigmatization of lesbians and gay men. In fact it would be wholly impossible to overestimate the extent to which the cultural deck is heterosexistly stacked. Lesbian poet Judy Grahn traces the term "bad" to its origins in the Anglo-Saxon "baedell" meaning "hermaphrodite." She remarks that the "very word used to judge whether something is to be acceptable or not acceptable is a word that once meant 'Gay'."

Profound unacceptability is certainly the message most lesbian and gay youth get about themselves. Because the essential years, which acclimate heterosexuals to the rituals of romantic relationship, become for young gays a torturous eternity of deception and facade. "What does this do to one's relationship with oneself?" asks Dr. Novick. "What does it do to one's relationship with others? . . . Society does not allow us the usual growth pattern of respectful relationship and the stigma makes sex a thing to be experienced secretly and briefly." One case in point is Brad, a PWA or person with Acquired Immune Deficiency Syndrome (AIDS).

AN EXAMPLE

Brad's family was comfortable and well-educated. Neither religious fanaticism nor overt neglect informed his upbringing. Yet his entirely ordinary, albeit somewhat privileged, midwestern U.S. childhood precipitated a life-long proclivity for truck stop and rest room sexual encounters.

Brad's siblings experienced the usual process of acquiring societal and relationship skills vis-à-vis "dating" in an atmosphere of reasonably comfortable interaction among family and friends. His sisters would often invite their boyfriends over. Congenial, if stilted, conversations would ensue, with the father's commenting about football or blustering about driving too fast. The brother's girlfriend was a fixture at family barbecues and frequently appeared for joint homework efforts.

Because he was gay, Brad's familial experience was the categoric opposite of his siblings'. While he maintained the obligatory heterosexual charade, at one point escorting a prospective nun to reduce the likelihood of romantic encounter, Brad's staggering isolation simply metastasized.

A WIDER VIEW

Statistics ground this perspective. For example, at Manhattan's Hetrick-Martin Institute for the Protection of Lesbian and Gay Youth, 21% of the clients have attempted suicide by the time they get to the facility. And the Institute's co-founders, Emery S. Hetrick, MD, and A. Damien Martin, EdD, report that every child involved cites "feeling totally alone with no one to talk to" as a reason for the attempt. The sickening depth of this isolation might be conveyed by the fact that some of the gay male and lesbian youngsters, who upon the circumstance of their suicide attempts had undergone treatment in non-gay facilities, *had not told their therapists about their sexual orientation.*

In other words, young people who had already tried to take their own lives were too afraid of the system's reaction to homosexuality to even bring up their sexual orientations. And Hetrick-Martin is not alone in its experience with such phenomena. A 1989 U.S. Department of Health and Human Services "Report of the Secretary's Task Force on Youth Suicide" placed lesbians and gay males at substantially increased risk, with some research showing suicide as the leading cause of death among sexual minority youth.

SILENCE

These findings are sure evidence that the darkness surrounding this major area of human experience is immediately fatal to no small number of U.S. children. But orientation was never even mentioned in Brad's family. That heterosexuality was presumed permeated every nuance of cultural, social, and educational discussion. No one knew (or knew that they knew) a homosexual. And while "faggot" (meaning "kindling," as derived from gay experience in burnings at the stake) was a playground epithet and "wimp" had its own grave implications, such subjects were simply beneath consideration in the respectability of adult middle class discourse.

Brief and quietly derisive allusion was once made to an "effeminate" acquaintance. It was concluded that, although he was "odd," nothing was really "wrong" (meaning gay) with the man. Thus Brad sustained the inescapable impression that his stirring young heart rendered him far more contemptible than anything his family might even discuss.

"How Nice!" sings feminist composer Kristin Lems:

> How Nice! Traditions have been carried.
> Now the family's in a flurry—
> Oh, it's such a happy ending!
> With rings and vows and showers
> They will certify their love,
> With presents from the relatives

And blessings from above.
But if both of them were women
Or if both of them were men,
Who would congratulate them then?

[Lems 80]

For a time Brad assumed, as do many gay youths, that he was the only "one" on the planet. Then, as boyhood cronies "out-grew" the practice of mutual sexual experimentation, Brad became more, not less, attracted to his own gender. Later, it was through the gossip of those same old friends that Brad learned of a much despised counterculture which continued its male-to-male interactions beyond childhood and anonymously.

A PATTERN

This subculture Brad discovered reflects a pattern that sometimes surfaces among young men who might, in a more supportive social context, "date" much as do their heterosexual peers. The taboo on emotional male-to-male relations encourages a separation of sexual and affectional capacities in those youth who are already wrestling with the incongruity of society's heterosexual expectations and their own emerging sexuality. Dr. Betty Berzon, a psychotherapist who is herself a lesbian, describes a stage on the path to gay identity wherein some males "keep sexual contacts free of emotional involvement and avoid repeated contacts with the same person."

The culture further compounds such patterns. Men are socialized to initiate rather than decline sexual adventure, leaving refusal to the discretion of women. But no such societal brakes are built into male/male relationships, and no non-sexual social environments are provided for these gay youth whose very existence the system refuses to acknowledge. Add to these elements the societal incentive for heterosexual facade (a permanent partner is an exceedingly difficult thing to hide), and a protracted no-strings sexual pattern is not an unlikely development.

It must be noted here that for many persons, of whatever orientation, enduring commitment is not a norm. Even in the rosy context of universal societal blessing, most recent heterosexual marriages end in divorce (New York *Daily News* 3/13/89). Nor does every commitment presume monogamy. The point is that such options are discouraged and indeed sometimes even precluded for persons so censured and vilified as gays.

Brad's romantic interests were channeled, thus, into a hitchhiking format: "I would stand, of an afternoon or evening, on the highway verge until someone 'wonderful' stopped." When mutuality permitted, sexual relations were consummated furtively and with great haste in the vehicle. Sometimes *no* preliminary syllables were exchanged, not even first names. After the encounter, Brad would ask to be dropped off nowhere near home, lest a neighbor observe the association.

LEARNING TO HIDE

"We've distanced ourselves from them [gays]," continued Dr. Novick in Bridgehampton, "and we may even hate them as much as straight people do. But now we may begin to hate ourselves — or our potential partners."

This distancing or "dissociation" often takes dramatic turns. Indeed such elaborate camouflage techniques are routinely adopted that Hetrick-Martin's Social Services Director, Joyce Hunter, MSW, reports with Dr. Martin that lesbian pregnancy and teen fatherhood are recurring problems among gay youth attempting to disguise their orientations.

Even more disturbingly, some closeted gays, to imply heterosexuality, join the ranks of murderous "queer bashers" for whom societal anti-gay rhetoric is as gasoline to a fire. In 1987 Nevada's 26-year-old Sean Patrick Flanagan murdered two men he perceived as gay. In a detailed statement, Flanagan explained that he hated his own homosexuality and thought he was "doing some good for our society." This particular outbreak of homophobia (fear of things gay) manifested three fatalities. On June 24, 1989 the *New York Times* reported Flanagan's execution for the murders.

As Dr. Martin notes in "Learning to Hide: The Socialization of the Gay Adolescent," the "dissociation stage may last late into adulthood, in fact may never be overcome, sometimes with tragic results." And in another offshoot of this obscuration, closeted gay officials have been not infrequently known to lead the fray against lesbian/gay civil rights.

FATALITIES

In 1989 Brad died of AIDS related complications. Perhaps the virus was passed along in the early years, when nothing could have been done to alert him. Or maybe he was exposed later in the epidemic, at a time when many could have protected themselves had the situation been publicized like a "Legionnaires' disease." But no such openness graces same-gender relationships, and Brad went the way of so many in the young gay male community.

He departed after 40 years in an atmosphere where every iota of the support with which society provides its heterosexual youth is a heat-seeking missile meticulously programmed for attack and destruction of the homoaffectional heart. Throughout his life, Brad's psyche had been routinely brutalized, vilified, and demoralized by church, school, Hollywood, and of course, the family, whose a priori exclusion distinguishes the gay minority from every other discrete group in being. That is, *even nuclear blood relatives are the agents of prejudice.*

Such is the bare surface of a crisis which, based on the percentage at which many health professionals estimate lesbian/gay-male incidence, must involve at least 10% of this country's youth. This is the crisis which Dr. Novick attributes to the "deepest of all social flaws — to value the macho." And it is Dr. Novick's profound thesis that, while the phenomenon of pervasive heterosexism has always been psychologically devastating, one must now regard "homophobia as a co-factor in the AIDS epidemic" by virtue of its impeding and preempting responsible relationships in a community where irresponsibility invites terminal illness: "They allow us no positive role models and then label us promiscuous and immoral. . . . "How bizarre," he mourned. "They work their evil on us then call us evil. How bizarre."

Brad's death was one casualty in a malicious societal routine which has, in the present accompaniment, turned genocidal. The homophobia which undermines gay relationships created a hotbed for sexually transmitted plague; and the government, in its coy reluctance to address matters homosexual, has resolutely exacerbated the situation. Under the tireless guidance of Senator Jesse Helms (R-NC), Congress actually defunded AIDS education programs in direct proportion to their effectiveness, i.e., their gay male specificity. As the Senator explains in the Congressional Record: "We have got to call a spade a spade and a perverted human being a perverted human being . . ." (S.14204 10/14/87).

That most gay men now practice a safer sex, which avoids the exchange of blood or semen, is almost entirely due to the efforts of the gay community itself, whose pioneer organizations like New York's Gay Men's Health Crisis mobilized a decade of exhaustive research and education. Of course, among the illiterate and non-English speaking, education is lagging and actively discouraged by Congress. Elected officials, it would seem, tend to regard pictorial sex-safety explanations as particularly "pornographic."

At other administrative levels, endless delays and political considerations have obstructed research and implementation of such programs as are authorized. The fact that the solvent dying, for the better part of the epidemic, have been flying to other countries for experimental treatments bears witness to a profound indifference in the U.S. bureaucracy. This disease has brought new meaning to feminist Holly Near's anthem: "We are a gentle angry people, and we are singing, Singing For Our Lives."

Yet, in many ways Brad was lucky as a youth. Because he was "closeted" (secretive) and able to "pass" for straight, he avoided a veritable gamut of pitfalls, including the heterosexual marriage "cure" and the incredibly destructive enforced reorientation attempts undergone by so many of our nation's young. Also, while some parents actually evict their lesbian or gay offspring, Brad's closet precluded this possibility. And Brad's encounter with police entrapment occurred late enough in life that he was able to avoid embarrassment in hometown media. For he had, like so many gays, fled his birthplace upon reaching majority. Consequently, it was a remote newspaper which reported his arrest by the police officer who had in fact *solicited him*.

But the biggest perk for the endless, invalidating, self-dividing deception of Brad's childhood was physical survival. For the Flanagan tragedy is but the tip of a very ugly national iceberg. At Hetrick-Martin, 40% of the clients have suffered physical attacks, including rape, as occasioned by their orientation [Hetrick 88].

In fact it was this persistent experience with peer-meted violence that inspired New York's Board of Education to co-initiate Hetrick-Martin's special off-site educational program. As the Institute's Joyce Hunter, herself a woman of color explains, many students experience the "double whammy" of racism and homophobia. For her role in co-founding the school program, Hunter received threats on the lives of her children (*New York Newsday* 9/15/88).

In 1988 the New York Governor's Task Force on Bias-Related Violence reported that "gays and lesbians may be the most victimized group in the nation." The finding will come as a surprise to some, as the report also found such crimes were "systematically under-reported by the press." Considering that cultural prejudice demands a substantial U.S. minority choose between physical safety and integrity of psyche, this is something less than a land of the free for lesbian and gay citizens.

PROSPECTS

The internalized societal-censure which impelled Brad to divorce his social and sexual lives made one-to-one relationships intensely precarious. Should his life have continued, however, he might have established the kind of long-term partnership he sometimes admired. A great many men and women of the gay community do form relationships every bit as stable as those of their heterosexual peers. And others, who have declined such relationships, arrive at them in time, a phenomenon Martin attributes to gays learning "at a later date those social interactions with peers that the heterosexual adolescent had the opportunity to learn during the teenage years." As he further explains: "Accepting homosexuality as normal would be optimal since it would make it possible for the adolescent to reach that fusion of sexuality and emotionality described as gay identity." Dr. Martin is not, however, overly optimistic in forecast: "For most, hiding and attempts to change are the strategies used to cope with their stigmatized status. Society does all in its power to reinforce these two strategies and thus prevents self-acceptance."

Thus is homophobia relentlessly sustained. Through it, fatalities persist in gay/lesbian youth suicide, anti-gay violence, and deterrent to respectful relationship in a community where responsibility is a life and death issue. Later chapters will explore sexual orientation more fully, along with some important new developments which can be brought to bear upon oppressive societal institutions, including the government. First, however, will come a lesbian viewpoint in the context of larger feminist thought.

CHAPTER 2

A LESBIAN PERSPECTIVE

"Then lesbians are the chosen people," goes the retort to a televangelist proclamation that AIDS is God's wrath upon gays. But, of course, the fact is that a plague, wreaking indiscriminate havoc abroad, found entré into a Western community whose insulated patterns simply confined it there for a time. This made gay males sacrificial laboratory specimens for a cataclysmic threat most officials and professionals chose to ignore. That people calling themselves spiritual leaders should feel free to vilify such a group is, in itself, an indictment of the country's longstanding indifference to a festering moralism. But arguing religion has for some time been considered "bad manners" in the United States.

INVISIBILITY

Of course, lesbians do, in fact, contract AIDS through various routes; no group is safe. But, incredibly, an entire decade of moralists remained completely oblivious to the relatively low AIDS incidence in lesbian women. Many observers simply did not make the jump that a sexually transmitted virus would not travel first to those least likely to be in sexual contact with the highest incidence group. Such incomprehension affords the clearest possible illustration of the insidious invisibility to which this society consigns its women and their sexualities. And some "fundamentalists," persons convinced that their own "moral" point of view is a norm ordained by God, are still now, into the 1990s, proclaiming that through Acquired Immune Deficiency Syndrome a male god is punishing homosexuality. These claims persist in spite of the disease's ravaging infants, Africans, heterosexuals, injection drug users, and the

10

blood-transfused, and in spite of the fact that half the country's gay people i.e., lesbians, are at the far end of the sexual transmission chain.

This sort of steadfast denial of gay women's existence actually provoked a language change in the '70s. The progressive vanguard adopted "lesbian" specifically to counter the subsumption of homosexual women under the male presumptive "gay."

EXPERIENCE

Unlikely as it may seem, the torturous experience of Brad's youth was probably more integrated than that of his typical lesbian counterparts. For men, after all, and especially white men, as was Brad, never are absent male privilege. Such prerogative implies a kind of celebration in sexual being, even when the orientation is unpopular. While the back street "cruising" arena provides for gay boys some awareness of like-oriented persons, young lesbians frequently have no relevant social network at all, sexual or otherwise. In fact, those young women who are self-aware enough to have identified their lesbianism could, until very recently, glean evidence of like-minded others only through scant literature in all of which tormented lesbians either perished or festered in relentless guilt.

One poet of this author's acquaintance sustained, at age 12, her very first ray of hope (that she wasn't the only "one" in the world) through notices about the 1962 film of Lillian Hellman's "The Children's Hour." A lesbian dies, of course (by suicide), but the reference sent the young woman tearing to a dictionary where she remembers reading "lesbian — the reputed sensuality of the people of Lesbos." This homophobic tautology told her nothing, but from the review itself it seemed that two women, somewhere, were believed to be lovers. In the face of that possibility, death was as nought.

Lesbian invisibility reflects society's resolute refusal to acknowledge sexual, male-free women in its midst. The term "gay," probably a relic of England's street slang, is now a political entity, chosen by the activist community as descriptive of a *people* rather than of a *behavior* (as is "homosexual"). Yet the perception of gay "sex" versus non-gay "love" endures. A heterosexual with a mate's picture on the desk is apple pie itself, while a lesbian or gay man in the same circumstance is "flaunting sexuality." And since gays are perceived as sexual rather than romantic entities, and since women are not allowed to be sexual entities, gay women, i.e., lesbians, for many people, simply do not exist.

THE LARGER NEGATION

The subsumption of women has troubled generations of United States citizens, from Abigail Adams' polite entreaty in 1776 that the Constitutional framers "remember the ladies" to the half million people in the 1989 Washington march for abortion rights. Lesbian invisibility is but a spinoff of the deeply instilled sexual negation which deforms women in general. In "our" patriarchal situation, the manifestation of male genitalia occasions privilege, pride and self-esteem. "It's a boy!" still carries a subtle and mysterious weight. And while Brad, for instance, was disposed to know when he was "turned on" and by whom, such is not always the case for women — a state of affairs which same-gender orientation can only aggravate.

For example, clinical psychologist Dr. Julia Heiman reports a test wherein 42% of women denied being sexually excited even as vasocongestion readings confirmed physiological arousal. In the same study, not a single man (0%) was unaware of his sexual response. Dr. Patricia Morokoff of the University of Rhode Island's Psychology Department, explains this phenomenon in terms of females having been "taught to restrict knowledge of their genitals and genital responses."

Heiman's research indicated further that arousal unawareness was most pronounced in the absence of "social validation" for "physical response." Morokoff continues: "Society presents an ambivalent message to women about sex: It is desirable to be sexually responsive with one's partner, but it is not desirable to be interested in sex for gratification of one's own sexual needs." She continued: "One way out of this double-bind is physiological response without awareness of arousal."

So some women don't know when they're "turned on"; and the

situation is most pronounced in the absence of social approval. Considering then, that such societal validation is conspicuously absent for the erotic choices of homosexual people, this author wonders: to what extent do how many women simply not recognize their lesbian orientations?

Findings about women's unnoticed physical arousal certainly imply that the "dissociation" or distancing from self which sometimes accompanies gays well into adulthood would have different ramifications in lesbians than in gay men. For while males might deny the emotionality of their relationships, women tend more to reject physical content. As Dr. Betty Berzon points out, the stage of development in which some gay males "keep sexual contacts free of emotional involvement" parallels a phase where females may "keep relationships with women strictly nonsexual, no matter how emotionally involving they are."

NUMBERS

The 1953 Kinsey report showed 13% of women as against 37% of males with at least one orgasmic adult homosexual experience and "half to a third" as many women as men "who were, in any age period, primarily or exclusively homosexual." Ten percent has become the ballpark presumption for exclusive or predominant lesbian/gay-male incidence, with a greater bisexuality presumed among the women. However, a comprehensive 1978 study, commissioned by the National Institute of Mental Health, suggested to researchers Bell and Weinberg that "the lesbians' greater heterosexuality simply reflects a history of accommodation to males in a sexual context or of conformity to societal expectations." So it may be that, in any count, there are more lesbians than meet the eye. Examples of late bloomers are easy to come by in the community:

INTERVIEWS

A doctor of psychology and former lawyer, Taylor says her orientation defined itself at age 41, six months after she began a recovery from alcoholism. She describes herself as having been "numbed out" since she began using alcohol at age 16. She "emotionally sleepwalked" through a decade of marriage wherein the man became sexually dysfunctional very early. She believes alcohol "veiled the orientation," and when the veil was removed "a lesbian was there." She maintains that "the Catholicism had a great deal to do with the need to numb out." She saw these forces "operating in retrospect" and was not in any sense conscious of her orientation which is today, as she explains it, "self defining."

A Matriarchal Minister

For some contemporary feminists, lesbianism is actually a sociopolitical choice. Such is the case with Deborah Ann Light, a philanthropist and minister of matriarchal religions. Deborah's orientation "evolved" with maturation. As an adult she noticed "that the other adults were women." She believes an "innate bisexuality" gave her "freedom to choose an orientation" consistent with her feminist spirituality: "Appreciating the Diety as female makes it realistic to worship the feminine. The act of love is an act of worship—totally different, and attuned to totality . . . awesome." At the time of her emergence as a lesbian Deborah was 47.

It is important that such flexibility not be presumed for the majority of people. Many experience definitive or predominant orientations very early. Indeed, some of the women in Kinsey's 1953 study reported "specifically erotic responses to other females when they were as young as three and four." But bisexuals represent a large group, distinct from exclusive and predominant homosexuals or heterosexuals. And it is a tenet of many professionals that mutability in itself implies bisexuality. As psychiatrist Jean Munzer remarked in a 1989 interview with the author: "To the degree of its exclusivity, the orientation overrides social demands."

An Activist

Elizabeth Terry, a fundraiser and rights activist from Philadelphia, realized at age 12 that she was not interested in boys in such ways as were her friends. She fell in love at 17 and became involved with a young woman who denied that she was gay and who eventually ended the relationship to marry a man. Elizabeth attempted heterosexual relationships for a few years, emerging, with some relief, at 20 into lesbian society. An African American, she sees herself "thrice blessed" to be of color, a woman, and gay. In her words: "Each minority perspective brings its own unique awareness and every awareness is a blessing."

An Academic

Still other lesbians emerge and yet deny it. Rose Walton, EdD, experienced her orientation at 17. Although her sexual relationships were almost exclusively with women, she did not consciously acknowledge her lesbianism until age 33. She explained her personal life as "just happening to be in love with a particular person," those 16 odd years being something of a "fluke."

Rose now heads a department in the School of Allied Health Professions at the State University of New York, where she is open about her orientation, even at a media level. She says that the School and University's supportive administrations, along with Governor Mario Cuomo's executive order prohibiting anti-gay discrimination in state agencies, provided a comfortable climate for her "coming out" process. Rose enjoys a 13-year relationship with Marge Sherwin, a physical therapist.

WOMEN'S ROOTS

What motivates the dramatic repression of women's sexuality, lesbian or otherwise? Civilization itself, it would seem, for the tale begins with prehistory: "The differences in strength which now divide the sexes hardly existed in those days, and are now environmental rather than innate," writes Pulitzer prize winning historian Will Durant. He describes the early male's familial position as "superficial and incidental" to the "fundamental and supreme" female role. And he remarks upon the colossal workload of early woman, a pattern he views as an exploitation of her extraordinary strength (woman being "not yet an ornament"). But he presumes a "period of mother-right," born of women's economic (agricultural) leadership, which was eventually "wrested from them by the men."

June Stephenson, PhD, traces this progression in an expansive narrative, *Women's Roots*. With established archaeologic and anthropologic data for a camp base, she scouts out women's transformation of the art of food gathering into the science of cultivation. Isolating patriarchy in the relatively recent context of civilization, Stephenson explains that it was through the domestication of animals that the male role in procreation was discerned. This development precipitated the decline of women's autonomy as men became more and more interested in identifying and claiming their offspring along with livestock and produce. The consequence was a solidification of the family as a basic economic unit and the implementation of chastity requirements to ride herd on the human goods. Durant concurs: "the male now demanded [from women] that fidelity which he thought would enable him to pass on his accumulations to children presumably his own."

Stephenson writes that, to this end, "it became necessary to restrict women, to put women out-of-bounds to any other male. Rules about virginity and adultery were eventually written into the male-dominated religious dogma." Then, as Durant remarks: "The gods, who had been mostly feminine, became great bearded patriarchs, with such harems as ambitious men dreamed of in their solitude." The eventual attribution of sexual restrictions to a male god deified such inequities as adultery based solely on female marital status, "illegitimacy" as a stigma, and in short, the indefatigable patriarchal jihad against reproductive freedom which perseveres in today's theopolitical "right-to-life" movement. Then, as now, the bottom line was controlling women.

CONTROL

Implementation of this control, of course, required restrictions of farther reach than sexuality. Autonomy itself was suspect and, as "purity" became more and more in demand, women were induced to be less and less capable of "preserving" it. For example, the "fashion" limiting upper body strength has, through millennia of "natural" selection, become a biologically as well as culturally enforced assault on women's innate capacity.

This weakening agency has the added feature of necessitating "protection" for the ever present attacks on women's persons. Compounded assault is imposed by the inculcation of "shame" regarding women's sexuality, so that rape becomes more than physical violence and produces a "guilt" so enduring that most such crimes are not even reported to the "protectors."

The purity-weakness pedestal in turn invites assault by males socialized to aggression. As was pointed out in a May 16, 1989 *New York Times* opinion column, anthropological studies have shown that "an ideology of male toughness" breeds rape-prone societies while "rape-free" societies encourage full female economic and political participation with "male involvement in child-rearing." Jane C. Hood, associate professor of sociology at the University of New Mexico, went on to say that a campaign to prevent assaults on women should encourage paternity-leave and gender equality in the work place.

The occasion for Professor Hood's remarks was a particularly violent teen gang rape of a young woman in New York's Central Park. On the same day, there appeared another *Times* column by actor Ned Beatty, who portrayed a rape victim in the movie "Deliverance." A subject of constant harassment about the scene, Beatty remarks on men's refusal to identify with the victim: "If we felt we could truly be victims of rape, that fear would be a better deterrent than the death penalty."

THE DRESS CODE

"The pedestal is the pits" goes the old feminist slogan. For pedestalization controls women — from the bride's white dress to the "59¢ dollar" (another feminist slogan now trending slightly upward) she'll earn if she works outside the home. Such control implies mechanical as well as biological debilitation. So most women go through life hobbled by costume, in the sense that it is almost impossible for a two-legged being (let alone a two-legged child) to maneuver freely in a dress or skirt, especially when "fashions" are short. One cannot, without risk of underwear exposure, mount a bike, sit without cutting off circulation, or for that matter walk over a hot air register. For children, this dress requirement has actually been government enforced to the degree of its implementation in public schools, education being a state mandated experience in the U.S.

This particular violation of young women's autonomy has been, to some extent, overturned by the civil disobedience of youngsters whose parents were feminist enough to permit such demonstrations. When New York City's Mayor Edward Koch's support of "gender appropriate" public school uniforms threatened to reinstitutionalize the sexist dress code, one veteran of the 1970s "dress wars" reminded His Honor that the action violated a significant increment in feminist progress. "Nearly a generation of schoolgirls," wrote Kathleen Condon to the October 24, 1988 *New York Times*, has "been able to walk to school through snow in relative warmth, slide into home plate without skinned knees, and dangle upside down from monkeybars without the worry that boys are eyeing their underwear." She explained that "the right of girls to wear pants to school was hard won, and had real meaning for the budding feminists who waged the struggle."

Double Standards

Men's having commandeered the practical garments also enforces gender caste. The stigmatic quality is evidenced by the curiosity that males are "ridiculous" in dresses while women in pants are simply "under-dressed" for many common occasions. So men, even formally, can get away with more serviceable garments while womanhood demands flimsy, unsubstantial, decorative apparel which by now carries an almost genetic reminder of inferior status.

Of course, there are many women (and some men too) who truly enjoy the most ethereal of garments. The political problem arises only insofar as hierarchal costume is *mandated*, that is, unavoidable for one gender and unavailable to the other.

Indeed, the deathless stereotype of dykely fashion trashing is soundly refuted by contemporary lesbians, many of whom are worthy of the glossiest magazines. But then, great numbers of lesbian school teachers, models, principals, journalists etc. have always looked traditionally fashionable. It's just that no one knew they were lesbians. And when almost no lesbians were "out" (of the closet), the few brave ones who were tended least to respect patriarchal traditions, aesthetic or otherwise.

For some years now, a heated dialogue has transpired between the '60s academics-type feminists of comfortable dress, and the "lifestyle" lesbian executives and professionals of more classic fashion. The subversion of traditional seductivity by the latter was patiently explained to the author by gay rights activist, Marie Manion, who once marched in a pride parade with a "lipstick lesbians" placard: "If skirts are designed for male accessibility, then they also facilitate female accessibility."

The Cinderella Syndrome

Nowhere is "dress code" hobbling more dramatic than vis-à-vis female footwear. In a brilliant chapter on footbinding, Doctor of theology and philosophy Mary Daly describes the 1,000 year "custom" which, in service of the Eastern male's erotic penchant for female dependence and immobility, literally disabled millions of Chinese women. This savage fetish, which mutilated female feet into useless stumps, was in the interest of "purity" (not being able to run around) and "fashion" with incentives like "marriageability" offsetting the fact that one was unable to flee, for example, an attacker.

The Western male, being similarly disposed, controls the economy by reserving the best jobs for himself while women have access to a full value dollar only through social associations with men who like high heels. Then, to attain even the lower paying jobs, women must wobble on spikes, gingerly avoiding grates, doubly vulnerable in terms of at risk pantyhose, and, as Daly puts it "painfully smiling" and "physically and emotionally unsteady." Perhaps apropos is another old movement alert to the effect that whatever dance Fred Astair did, Ginger Rogers had to execute backwards and in high heels. Daly points up sexism's global connections with a reminder that "Cinderella," whose shortness of foot wins the coveted prize of princely attention, is of Eastern origin.

Glimmerings

Inroads are, of course, being made. A succinct analysis of the situation appeared in the extremely unlikely context of a *New York Times* Russell Baker column (2/18/89): "In the past few years the city has started walking faster than ever because New York women have given up wearing fancy shoes on the street and now lope along as swiftly as General William Tecumseh Sherman's long-legged Army of the West." Describing the new facile footwear as "uglifying" Mr. Baker continues: "The women usually change into unsensible shoes when they get to work. Why not a sensible dress shoe for women? Pedisexism, I guess." Guess so, Russ.

SUBTLER RESTRAINTS

But along with physical impairments come the psychological devices. As Dr. Leslie Brody, a psychologist at Boston University, reports, a comprehensive review of the data strongly suggests that "parents socialize the emotional development of boys and girls differently. . . . thus contributing to differences in males' and females' emotional functioning."

Travel in these emotional territories is, in many ways, distinct from the more objective feminism which steers female children to chemistry sets and expands boys' options into women's traditional domain. For emotional patterning represents the most subtle underpinnings of pink and blue, the forgotten agenda in whose service people growl at male babies and coo falsetto at the pinks. It informs the tones in which conversation is conducted and the topics emphasized. It involves a routine, ritualized brainwashing which begins sometimes before the baby itself is bathed. And it manifests as a polarity whose extremes are warlike, now nuclear men, and depression-prone, victimized women receiving financial and social approval in proportion to the degree of their suppression.

In both genders, emotions, essential to balanced experience and expression, are re-routed respective to genitalia. The July 1, 1989 *New York Times* reported that now many education researchers even attribute what's left of the scholastic "gender gap" (a variant, previously presumed "biological," in males' and females' fields of excellence) to self-confidence disturbed by role indoctrination.

SUGAR AND SPICE

If any specific aspect of women's experience rivals sexuality for such be-gendered re-circuiting, it is her anger. Like "inappropriate" sexual arousal, female anger goes unnoticed, unreported, unrecognized, redefined and smiled through. Dr. Brody explains that while girls are socialized to "fear," parents indoctrinate boys to "anger" through emphasis in story telling and acceptance of expression. And adaptation of females to "their lower status and power relative to men" demands "the minimization of anger, and the emotional expression of vulnerability and weakness.

As women we are angry. Some of us know it and some of us don't. But we are turning it against ourselves in depression, resentment, and illness. Men, angry at tyranny, dumped shiploads of tea into the ocean, started a terrific war, and are this country's heroes. Yet suffragists were "shrill," feminists wishing to control their own bodies are "strident," and visible lesbian activists are "mannish." Anger is simply not tolerated in women. A level of communication which registers as "effective" in men computes, among both men and women, as "anger" when it manifests in women. And giggle quotas are such that women are often cited for anger that was neither expressed nor intended. Unsmiling delivery is "hostile" — except in men where it is a norm.

The author is a long time participant in an alcoholism recovery program which tends to decry anger as a "do not." But this program was developed by men, in whom anger is instilled as a *cover* for genuine sensibilities. In women, the exact opposite is true. Here anger is often a *clue* to genuine sensibility. It is sometimes the first bread crumb on the long trail back to integration and sanity. And while anger may signal a dangerous period, during which additional safeguards against drinking should be maintained, it should not be further contorted into more of the depression and self-deprecation which are so common among alcoholic women.

Anger is a valid, validating and vital emotion. It validates the agent by its reality and it validates the recipient through earnest recognition. As Dr. Beverly Harrison, a professor of Christian Social Ethics at Manhattan's Union Theological Seminary, puts it:

"Anger expressed directly is a mode of taking the other seriously, of caring."

THERAPIES

Indeed taking anger seriously is essential to *A Feminist Position on Mental Health*. In a book by that title, Dr. Mary Ballou and Nancy W. Gabalac, MEd, stress the centrality of anger and other emotions in feminist psychotherapy. They explain that because woman is "a person who has been told what to feel and what she must not feel until her perceptions have become distorted, she now must learn to recognize her own data and her own experiences which are uncontaminated by the power systems bias."

Nowhere is this more pertinent than among lesbians. In present society, the artifices which have grown up around gender are the very *format* for identity. Lesbians, demeaned by mandated invisibility, are as women impugned for resisting the straightjacket of "ladyhood" and as gays impugned for immunity to a heterosexist "norm" which exists nowhere in nature. And, of course, lesbians of color experience a full complement of sexism, heterosexism, and racism, none of which proceed exclusively from the non-gay community.

The patriarchal context has necessitated a "feminist psychotherapy," which validates women's anger and experience, often turning personal recovery political, with some women risking employment and personal safety in the interest of visibility and network. Through such actions, feminists hope to impel the dominant society toward inclusion of its non-males, its non-whites, its non-heterosexuals, its Jews, its people with disabling conditions, and its otherwise atypical citizens.

The truth is that failed patriarchal indoctrinations give rise to healthy persons whose social orientations do in fact reflect their sexual orientations (hetero-, homo-, or bisexual), and whose gender "conformity," or lack of it, reflects their actual being. The '60s generation recoiled at the office cubicle and the war in Vietnam, effecting, in its rebellion, an expansive atmosphere conducive to social progress for women and gay men. The civil rights movement paved miles of bumpy road for feminists. To this day, a great many black men are strong legislative and political proponents of women's rights, reproductive freedom and lesbian/gay civil rights. And although the anti-war and early civil rights movements largely featured their men, feminists emerging from them carry on the fight against that chauvinism which so informs militarism and racism. But same-gender orientation is still somewhat beyond the social pale. And as long as this state of affairs persists, "lesbian" will remain an "epithet" to "threaten" any women whose identities exceed societal prescriptions.

In the personal/political adventure of feminist resolution to such conflicts, armament is essential and the best provision is information with which to debunk three odd millennia of patriarchal presumption. To this end do the following chapters address themselves in an exploration of evolving psychological, political, theological, and eventually metaphysical perspectives.

CHAPTER 3

PSYCHOLOGY

"There are no medical aspects to homosexuality." Clinical psychologist and Presbyterian minister James Harrison, PhD, had been asked to discuss the psychological, sociological, and medical aspects of homosexuality at Queens College, CUNY on October 19, 1985. He began his remarks with a flat statement: "There are no medical aspects to homosexuality. The only issue that medicine has to deal with concerning homosexuality is the need to rectify the profound misinformation that most physicians have about it."

The persistence of a "medicalized" model for homosexuality is a function of the general sexism pervading mental health fields. For the cultural presumption of autonomy as the exclusive province of men gained psychological as well as biological credence. To the degree that homosexuals frightened the horses of this "natural order," were they medically impugned.

FREUD'S LEGACY

Historic sexism was perhaps at its most exaggerated in the Victorian era. And it was this paradigm that Austrian psychiatrist Sigmund Freud (1856-1939) freeze-framed in his "fatherhood" of what was to become for decades the bottom line in mental health orthodoxy, psychoanalysis. Although Freud brought sex per se out of the closet, certainly a refreshing development in the context, much misogyny pervaded his legacy.

For Freud, a masculine ideal entailed the repudiation of aspects "feminine." Anatomically disallowed such consummation, as Freud saw it, women's lives—healthy women's lives—were organized around "penis envy," under whose auspices they vicariously

24

appropriated bits of the masculinity prize. Of course, many feminists, some of them analysts themselves, wondered who would not conjure up some small degree of male emulation, whether in Victorian Vienna or elsewhere. After all, the male sex organ had become a sole criteria for personhood, privilege, and education in the context of a completely devalued women's terrain.

Yet, as Betty Friedan detailed in 1963's *The Feminine Mystique*, not only did the Freudian schematic pervade the health professions, but also was it hyped and hyperbolized by the media and pop culture into breakfast table conversation for this country's declared grassroots. So in 20th century U.S.A., just as opportunities for higher education were beginning to provide some relief from the condescending Victorian "protectionism" of females, the faddish hawking of Freudian analysis redocumented the old, old business of men controlling women, this time as patently hip, avant garde, and grounded now in "modern science."

WOMEN AND MADNESS

A devastating prescription for human development was thus chiseled in the bedrock of orthodoxy. In 1972 Dr. Phyllis Chesler's *Women and Madness* decried the mental health field's routine institutionalization and narcotizing of women for such "psychoses" as independence, creativity, honestly expressed anger, and self preservation. Women's "health" itself implied a level of dependence considered pathological in men, with women who repossessed male provinces impugned to the exact extent of their autonomy.

In spite of Chesler's exposé and other cogent critiques, the bias Freud institutionalized endured. Over a decade later, in an overview of psychoanalysis and feminism, Dr. Jessica Benjamin, a psychoanalyst, was moved to remark: "The problem I have identified is that the predominant ideal, theory, and practice of autonomy in our culture is associated with the repudiation of the maternal and the feminine."

Today, psychoanalysis is only one of a great many psychological disciplines. And many practitioners with analytic backgrounds have proceeded far afield from traditional analysis. But because of the popularity the discipline itself gained among the general public, it is, in the business of debunking patriarchy, of some importance to examine psychoanalysis in a contemporary perspective, especially vis-à-vis lesbians and gay men.

Homophobia was intimated, rather than cemented, into psychoanalysis by its founder. And although an insidious Freudian anti-gay bias was presumed by latter day analysts, Freud himself wrote in 1905: "the exclusive interest of the man for the woman is also a problem requiring an explanation, and is not something that is self-evident."

LEWES ON FREUD

In a definitive and unprecedented historical overview of psychoanalysis and homosexuality (albeit male homosexuality), clinical psychologist Kenneth Lewes, PhD, documents the thesis "that the psychoanalytic bias against male homosexuals derives from an initial gynecophobic stance in psychoanalysis." He further submits "that the fear and denigration of women which hover at the perimeter of analytic discourse became displaced onto the theory of male homosexuality" [Lewes 88 p 21].

What's Good for the Goose . . .

In *The Psychoanalytic Theory of Male Homosexuality* Lewes disputes the premise that Freud thought male homosexuality disordered by virtue of its "narcissistic" object choice. Partner selection posited on resemblance to self, and a related affinity for "being loved" rather than "loving," were for Freud presumed *norms* in women. So Lewes argues that precisely because these dispositions characterized "half the race: the normal heterosexual female," they indeed "could not be considered inferior" [Lewes 88 p 74].

No Psychoanalytic "Cure"

And in 1920, Freud had asserted that "to undertake to convert a fully developed homosexual into a heterosexual is not more promising than to do the reverse." Recalling Freud's related belief that in the determination of sexual orientation inborn factors probably outweighed environmental ones, Lewes despairs that these immutable "preoedipal" elements were, without substantiation, turned into fair game for analytic "cure." He further decries the failures in discourse and compassion on this subject as "a stain on the history of psychoanalysis" [Lewes 88 p 121].

Citing Freud's persistent contention that bisexuality was innate in every being's constitution, Lewes explains that, in the central Freudian "Oedipus" mechanism (an interaction with the parents) all orientational outcomes are the results of "trauma," hence all are equally "normal." Freud's failure, Lewes writes, to enshrine a healthy homosexuality, was solely by dint of his *error* in grounding adult sexuality in the "act of procreation," which was for Freud "the central fact of human existence" [Lewes 88 pp 79-92].

Although Freud expected the *acquisition* of reproductive intent as a "social goal," Lewes recalls that: "The primacy of the genitals is a biological fact, but not whether an individual uses them for reproduction or pleasure or both." He goes on to assail the imposition of societal prescriptions onto psychoanalysis as founded in "ethics, politics and aesthetics" [Lewes 88 p 91].

Gay Analysts

An exclusion (which Freud had expressly opposed in 1921) of homosexuals from analytic training left articulation of the gay position even more foreclosed than was that of women, who were at least *represented* in the discipline. Concerning this, Lewes royally castigates the latter day analysts who demean gay contributions to analytic discourse [Lewes 88 p 240].

A final indictment proceeds from the profession's resolute refusal to acknowledge the significance of the 1948 Kinsey report which quite simply blew the rest of this country out of the water. Lewes sees this obtusity as evidence that "psychoanalytic thinking about homosexuality . . . had by this time become impervious to influence from outside psychoanalysis" [Lewes 88 p 138]. And rightly said, for if Freud had rendered sex mentionable, then Alfred C. Kinsey, the meticulous zoology professor, had made it evident there was more to mention than met the eye.

THE KINSEY REPORT

Kinsey's *Sexual Behavior in the Human Male* presented an orientation "continuum," with individuals reflecting a mix of homo- and heterosexuality. It was shown that, of the total white adult male population (this study so confined itself), 37% had "at least some overt homosexual experience to the point of orgasm" with 13% predominantly homosexual for at least 3 years, and another 13% reacting homoerotically without contacts. Kinsey considered his figures low for various reasons, among them that many married men with homosexual experience had avoided the survey. And he regarded the capacity to respond erotically to either gender as "basic in the species."

Kinsey also considered that choice of sexual partner had importance only insofar as society wished to dictate this matter. And he savaged the legal persecution of gay persons, exclaiming that "at least 13% of the male population . . . would have to be institutionalized and isolated, if all persons who were predominantly homosexual were to be handled in that way."

THE BREAKTHROUGH

As it happened, certain psychoanalysts, most notably Judd Marmor, MD, did understand homosexuals' perceived pathology as a function of the "cultural condemnation" rather than the orientation [Marmor 65]. But it was insight, not among the analysts, but in the larger mental health community's sociologists, psychologists, psychiatrists, and biologists which occasioned the American Psychiatric Association's eventual reform. And a vicious opposition was led by an analyst named Charles W. Socarides, MD, whose lifelong crusade against same-gender love as "demeaning and injurious to pride" remains an inexhaustible resource for contemporary anti-gay fundamentalists who discover in him a "scientist" as phobic as themselves. It is with this reactionary legacy in mind that Kenneth Lewes implores today's yet homophobic analytic community to admit evidence "from biology, on the one hand, and the social sciences, on the other" [Lewes 88 p 240].

In a *New York Times Book Review* (12/11/88) another very major voice in the discourse on orientation, UCLA professor of psychiatry and law Richard Green, MD, JD, praised Lewes for a "supurb synthesis, which will richly serve future scholars," but despaired of his insights' having any influence on the yet ossified analytic perspective: "Mr. Lewes remains a psychoanalyst and, believing that his profession has a unique value for the homosexual, yearns for a return to the noble spirit of Freud."

In 1973 the American Psychiatric Association removed homosexuality from the organization's list of mental disorders, concurrently deploring "all private and public discrimination against homosexuals in such areas as employment, housing, public accommodations" and further urging "the enactment of civil rights legislation at local, state, and federal levels that would insure homosexual citizens the same protections now guaranteed to others." The psychiatrists also recommended "the repeal of all legislation making criminal offenses of sexual acts performed by consenting adults in private."

DR. EVELYN HOOKER

Directly informing this decision were several developments including, most significantly, Dr. Evelyn Hooker's demonstrations through psychological profiles that the psychiatric community was unable to distinguish homosexuals from heterosexuals by any feature other than their orientation. Hooker's research with non-clinical subjects distinguished itself from earlier studies, which had involved persons seeking psychiatric help, a community among whom pristine mental health is not always a long suit. The findings, eventually incorporated in a National Institute of Mental Health Task Force on Homosexuality report, meant simply that homosexuality did not imply pathology.

The psychiatrists' policy was soon adopted by most mental health clinicians. The American Psychological Association concurred in 1975 "to oppose discrimination of homosexuals and to support the recent action by the American Psychiatric Association which removed homosexuality from that association's list of mental disorders."

These awakenings represented a life and death breakthrough in the lesbian/gay-male community's ongoing quest for human status in the United States. Indeed the medicalization phenomenon had been, in some ways, worse than the burnings that went before. Here, the bad people whom society would make good had become the sick people whom psychiatry would make well—this through all formidable manner of "treatment." Incarceration in mental facilities replaced incarceration in prisons. "Conversions" were attempted with legion failures and many of the good doctors despaired of a "cure," in some cases actively striving for sexual dysfunction.

SECOND CLASS STATUS

A compilation of such violations appears in Dr. Charles Silverstein's parents' guide to homosexuality *A Family Matter*. Lobotomies and anti-androgens were administered, gravely endangering "patients'" lives [Silverstein 77 pp 167-9] while "behaviorists," several of whom later declared that long-term orientation changes were not possible, practiced electric shock aversion therapy to separate gays from their same-gender partners. Resistance to such treatment was routinely reprimanded, returning the gay "patients" to their earlier status of "bad" persons who refused to let the "good" psychiatrist "cure" their "sickness."

Almost as destructive is the psychological epithet "immature," which selectively sanctions gays (as opposed to Roman Catholic priests and birth controllers) for their non-reproductive direction. This designation is particularly smarmy in that it implies true adult identity somehow eludes lesbians and gay men. (At least "evil" had some character.) And it should be argued that lesbians and gay men, having forged identities in completely hostile environments, are often hugely more self aware than are their non-gay counterparts.

Nor are same-sexers alone as a category upon whom health practitioners have visited their vilification. The 19th century medical climate was formally hostile to sexual gratification per se, as experienced by any other than men, heterosexually. As Silverstein reports, women, having been convinced that sexual response itself was morally and physically dangerous, sometimes underwent cliterodectomies to clear up "mental disorders" like orgasm, masturbation, and interest in contraception [Silverstein 77 p 166]. And the products we know today as graham crackers and corn flakes were originally developed by the evangelical Reverend Sylvester Graham and a John Harvey Kellogg, MD, in their bizarre conviction that the substitution of nuts and grains for meat foods would discourage masturbation in children [Money 85]. It seemed that the gentlemen hoped, through their products, to avert such pitfalls as "masturbatory insanity" and an analogously induced liver damage.

POOF!

If the first Kinsey report had burst this pseudomedical dirigible, then Kinsey on females, in 1953, atomized the considerable hot gas which had held it up. The women's "half to a third" of the male homosexual incidence was not as dramatic as the men's scores. But *Sexual Behavior in the Human Female* simply cannibalized such bastions of orthodoxy as the exclusive normalcy of sex for reproduction: "Biologists and psychologists who have accepted the doctrine that the only natural function of sex is reproduction, have simply ignored the existence of sexual activity which is not reproductive." Also, the penis was earnestly devalued by a passage on the "relative unimportance of the vagina as a center of erotic stimulation." As Kinsey put it: "Freud recognized that the clitoris is highly sensitive and the vagina insensitive in the younger female, but he contended that psychosexual maturation involved a subordination of clitoral reactions and a development of sensitivity within the vagina itself." Kinsey fairly screams: "but there are no anatomic data to indicate that such a physical transformation has ever been observed or is possible."

Kinsey on Freud

Taking the old Viennese psychiatrist further to task, the zoologist persists: "This question is one of considerable importance because much of the literature and many of the clinicians, including psychoanalysts and some of the clinical psychologists and marriage counselors, have expended considerable effort trying to teach their patients to transfer 'clitoral responses' into 'vaginal responses.' Some hundreds of the women in our own study and many thousands of the patients of certain clinicians have consequently been much disturbed by their failure to accomplish this biologic impossibility." This salvaging of the clitoris had rather broad implications for the sexual autonomy of women, as a predominant external sensitivity also called to mind a more active, versus receptive, female sexual capacity.

And the good professor also conducted a comparison of women in 5-year heterosexual vs. homosexual relationships wherein the higher frequencies of lesbians' orgasms were attributed to "considerable psychologic stimulation" and a presumed better understanding of female anatomy. One can only try to recapture the interest with which Eisenhower's United States read: "It is, of course, quite possible for males to learn enough about female sexual responses to make their heterosexual contacts as effective as females make most homosexual contacts."

So penile stimulation was in ways incidental to female orgasm, and also paled somewhat in dykely competition. What's more, lesbian antelope had been discovered (!) along with same-sex contact among "practically every species of mammal." Then how "unnatural" could it be? Such contacts did, it seems, "occur with considerable frequency" and "in such widely separated species as rats, mice, hamsters, guinea pigs, rabbits, porcupines, marten, cattle . . . goats, horses, pigs, lions, sheep, monkeys, and chimpanzees."

BELL ET AL.

Later studies countered a wide range of popular and professional misconceptions, some showing that neither parents nor society had much effect on sexual orientation. The qualities which emerge as sexual orientation are established very early in life, usually by the age of five [Money 80]. And research by Dr. Alan Bell et al. indicated that "homosexuality is as deeply ingrained as heterosexuality, so that the differences in behaviors or social experiences of prehomosexual boys and girls and their preheterosexual counterparts reflect or express, rather than cause, their eventual homosexual preference." This comprehensive 1981 study of 1,500 non-clinical subjects went on to show that: "No particular phenomenon of family life can be singled out . . . as especially consequential for either homosexual or heterosexual development" [Bell 81 pp 190-1]. And contrary to prevailing myth, gay people lacked neither heterosexual opportunity nor experience but rather registered such encounters as superficial and ungratifying [Bell 81 p 113]. Nor were gay adults, by any estimation, the product of pederastic childhood experiences: "the popular stereotype that homosexuality results when a boy is 'seduced' by an older male or a girl by an older female is not supported by our data" [Bell 81 p 185].

Findings concerning a high incidence of "gender nonconformity" in both lesbians and gay men [Bell 81 p 188] led the researchers to speculate that such atypical behavior might actually be the cause rather than the consequence of the "disturbed family relationships" [Bell 81 p 218] found in "tenuous" connection with the development of homosexuality [Bell 81 p 184]. And with respect to general familial influences, the writers summarized that orientation, heterosexual or homosexual, "is a pattern of feelings and reactions within the child that cannot be traced back to a single social or psychological root; indeed, homosexuality may arise from a biological precursor (as do left-handedness and allergies, for example) that parents cannot control" [Bell 81 p 192].

DR. MONEY

This allusion concurs with other distinguished opinion. In 1976 a quintessential authority in the field of sexology, John Money (Professor of Medical Psychology and Professor of Pediatrics, Emeritus at The Johns Hopkins Hospital and School of Medicine) issued the following statement to the House Judiciary Committee in Annapolis, Maryland: "Some people are left-handed, some ambidextrous, and some right-handed. The cause is not fully explainable, though there does appear to be an innate plus a learned component. The same applies to homosexuality, bisexuality, and heterosexuality." Imploring the State of Maryland to protect its lesbian and gay male citizens, Dr. Money explained that "it is not possible to force a change from homosexuality to bisexuality, any more than it is possible to force a heterosexual person into becoming a homosexual."

DR. GREEN

Dr. Richard Green's extensive study of gender nonconforming boys, *The "Sissy Boy Syndrome" and the Development of Homosexuality*, showed that neither parental intent nor specific psychiatric treatment obstructed the emergence of same-gender orientation in the children. Some of Green's subjects were treated by psychologists who hoped to avert the development of adult homosexuality which frequently accompanies pronounced gender atypicality. The efforts did not "interrupt the progression from 'feminine' boy to homosexual or bisexual man" and "the results, showing no major impact of treatment on sexual orientation" suggested also that the parental concern, which had occasioned such specific therapy, "did not operate to influence later sexuality" [Green 87 p 318].

What did happen was that many of Green's subjects were helped to avert or handle some of the merciless physical and verbal bashings such children experience at the hands of their more conventional peers. Green's conscientious advice to colleagues less versed in this area is that: "Reduction of conflict and stigma will remain viable treatment goals until society evolves to the point of accommodating greater latitude in the boyhood expression of currently 'sex-typed' behaviors" [Green 87 p 319].

THE REORIENTATION FALLACY

Many contemporary therapists share the view of Dr. Richard A. Isay, Clinical Professor of Psychiatry at Cornell Medical College, that it is "not possible, even at an early age, that you can do anything to alter sexual orientation" and that "the attempt to do that is going to damage the self-esteem of the child" (*USA Today* 3/1/89). This is not to say that spontaneous or apparent changes don't occur in either direction. As was mentioned in the previous chapter, bisexuals, people from the middle of the homo-hetero continuum, are more likely to be able to "choose" conformity to heterosexual ultimata. But such voluntary versatility defies the centrality and immediacy with which most orientations emerge. As Alan Bell et al. remarked of the 1981 Kinsey Institute publication: "Although we

have entitled our present work *Sexual Preference,* we do not mean
to imply that a given sexual orientation is the result of a conscious
decision . . .'' [Bell 81 p 222].

So an important question to ask about ''reorientation'' claims is
whether the subjects were predominantly or exclusively gay to begin with, or whether they emerged from the rather large body of
individuals who experience themselves bisexually. Another excellent line of inquiry is to determine what magnitude of dogma was
being brought to bear upon an individual to behave heterosexually
and to proclaim reorientation. Pressure to religious conformity has
been known to induce everything from mass marriage to mass suicide.

''Ex-gay'' is a political term devised by fundamentalists to imply
that their dogmata have altered orientation. A ''documentation''
(by Pattison and Pattison) of one such scenario cites as evidence of
movement from ''exclusive homosexuality to exclusive heterosexuality'' an example involving eleven young men, six of whom had
wed, one remarrying a former wife. Heterosexual relations were not
discussed and three of the group converting from ''exclusive homosexuality'' were formerly *self-described* bisexuals. Of the eleven,
all were ashamed and guilty about their same-gender contacts, all
had found their homosexual experiences disappointing and ''emotionally unfulfilling'' (a characteristic most gays experience in their
heterosexual but certainly not their same-gender encounters), and
all ''wanted to change to heterosexuality as a religious responsibility.'' That gay fantasies, dreams, and in one case experience continued in the subjects was dismissed as typically heterosexual for
some, but in others was a neurotic content which their heterosexuality endured. The heterosexual successes of the other five were discovered in that they all ''looked forward to marriage,'' having been
induced to celibacy by the pentacostals. ''Three were actively dating,'' the report explains. Hetrick and Martin, of the institute which
so often picks up the endoctrinational pieces of children forced by
parents and counselors into such religious environments, consum-
mately assail them as ''celibacy cults'' which encourage denial and
dissociation.

AN ETHICAL MANDATE

Of course, discomfort with one's sexuality (psychiatrically termed "ego dystonic" orientation) is almost always socially inspired. Part of the whole cloth of gay as well as non-gay orientation is that it is a core identity element which is badly violated by injunction to change. It is, says Dr. Harold Kooden (an openly gay Manhattan psychotherapist), precisely because of the internalized opprobrium that the expression of a desire to change is extremely suspect and is very likely to reflect "a social fantasy at odds with the orientation. The therapist has an absolute mandate," Kooden continues (in a 1989 interview with the author) "to find out to what degree the difficulties are a function of the culture. The ethical treatment is to thoroughly examine the conventional fantasy and determine to what extent it is predicated upon a desire for approval." He adds that an extremely important aspect of mental health is the patient's contact with gay peers, who help to neutralize society's negative input. Considering the isolation consistently specified by gay youth as precipitating suicide attempts, it would seem impossible to overstress the importance of such non sexualized socialization.

TRANSEXUALITY

Would my conflict have been so bitter if I had been born now, when the gender line is so much less rigid? If society had allowed me to live in the gender I preferred, would I have bothered to change sex?

Jan Morris 1974

The philosophy of enforced heterosexuality breeds not only suicide ideation but also transsexualism, a discomfort with being in one's own body. Hetrick and Martin report that some young gay boys are unable to conceive of themselves as men and try to become women. Joyce Hunter and A. Damien Martin relate an account of a young male whose "cultural belief that gay men are not male and therefore must be female" was motivating his acquisition of illegal hormone injections to develop breasts.

Also, Green's interviews revealed that some of the boys who had deemed homosexual relationships so taboo as to be inconceivable were in fact relieved of their gender discontent through the eventual acceptance of their homosexual orientations. One such young man said: "Maybe it was because I had always been homosexual, and I thought in order to have a sexual relationship with men, back then, I'd have to be a woman. I couldn't be a man and have a sexual relationship with a man. Maybe then, you know, I never thought about men making love to men. I always thought I had to be a woman to have a relationship with a man" [Green 87 p 367]. Another boy said, after his emergence as gay, that as a child his "effeminacy . . . and playing the role of women came less from a real desire to be a woman than from the fact that knowing, on a certain level, that I was gay all my life, and having no acceptable model or image of how to be a man and be gay, and feeling well, if I want men, if I'm attracted to men, then I have to be a woman" [Green 87 p 188].

Transexuality has meaning primarily within a heterosexist and begendered context. If one could dress, speak, and act as one wished, and freely, with societal survival, marry a person one was able to love, it may well be that fewer transsexuals would require hormonal and surgical reassignment. It is the blind acceptance of sex categories as *objectively valid* that so interferes with the experienced identities of the atypical. Of course, information about viable and respectful same-gender relationships can sometimes effect a return to sanity for these often deeply disturbed transsexual youth. But relevant education occasions such religious and governmental censorship that it almost always eludes those who need it most.

FOR YOUR OWN GOOD

"Well meaning" parents try to persuade their offspring, with variations on the race/religion argument, that people should pair off in accordance with societal expectations "for their own sakes." But while it is possible, if bigoted, to seek out marriageable Catholics,

Jews, Blacks, Asians, Caucasians, etc., what lesbian and gay male children hear is that they must be forever alone. There is certainly no one in their "appropriate" categories who would be in any way adequate. And should gay persons be dispossessed of this truth through therapy or religion, what manifests is a prescription for divorce, deception, and anonymous sex, not to mention the callous disregard for unsuspecting non-gay partners who are duped into wasting vast periods of their lives undertaking impossible orientation "cures."

An analogy for "voluntary" orientation treatment may perhaps be seen in India's suttee where widows, some of them half a century their husbands' juniors, "chose" either prostitution, abject poverty, or live incineration at the funeral pyre of their deceased spouses. Through this immediately fatal situation the conflation of "voluntary" and "enforced" are apparent. Perhaps AIDS will deliver gays such a focus in the contemporary U.S.

Persons wishing to "take on" the psychologically homophobic may consider honing in on these points for argument:

- Orientation is established by the age of 5.
- Same gender orientation does not connote pathology.
- Same gender orientation does not connote immaturity.
- Same gender orientation is entirely natural and occurs in all species.
- Attempts at reorientation are non-productive.
- Attempts at reorientation reinforce an already extremely destructive opprobrium.
- The vast majority of gay people were raised by heterosexuals whose universally reinforced indoctrination has not effected a heterosexual orientation in their offspring.

HOMOPHOBIA

While homosexuality is not pathological, homophobia is. Lesbians and gay men are extremely frequent victims of bias-related violence, as well as job and housing discrimination. So the overwhelming majority of men and women in the gay community feel obliged to maintain an elaborate and exhausting subterfuge of closeted living in order to protect their employment, their homes, and their lives.

Many lesbians and gay men hide not only from the outside world, but also from friends and families. Great numbers feel obliged to continually monitor behavior, reinforcing, throughout the decades, a self-image of unmentionable defect. And all gays, all of us, whether we honor it or not, encounter a lifelong societal demand to pretend to be someone else — often as the price of survival.

"Why am I gay" is a meaningless inquiry. As Dr. Marmor wrote in 1965: "'ambisexuality' is the biologic norm," not heterosexuality. He added that "exclusive heterosexuality is a culturally imposed restriction." In 1988 John Money explained that "in all species, the differentiation of sexual orientation . . . is a sequential process" operating prenatally "under the aegis of brain hormonalization" and continuing "postnatally under the aegis of the senses and social communication and learning." But this "biologic" issue is of more than just passing psychological curiosity. For some existing minority status protections are *triggered* by characteristics considered innate through biological basis (e.g., ethnicity).

Dr. Richard Green, on the April 12, 1989 Phil Donahue show, summarily quipped that "the answer to the question 'is homosexuality learned or inborn?' is 'yes.'" And he took the occasion of the Lewes book review (discussed previously) to royally upbraid those psychoanalysts who frustrate the gay civil rights Freud supported by "defensively contradicting the growing evidence for innate contributions to homosexuality."

CIVIL LIBERTIES

It is, of course, just plain wrong to postulate rights solely on innateness. Nor are all existing liberties so predicated. Religion is certainly an acquired trait, yet civil rights statutes specifically protect fundamentalists opposing rights for the gays whom they insist have a "choice" to be more like them through religious conversion. All of which deliberation is to soundly miss the point, which is: Whether or not the determinants of orientation are inborn or ac-

quired, why is the United States government in the business of telling anyone whom to love?

The political tracking of "natural vs. nurtural" orientational an-
tecedents will persevere because still menacing is the cavalier perspective that "acquired" characteristics are mutable and could/
should be changed. But this industrious count of angels upon pin
heads may have dangerous implications, in that *any* "cause" seized
upon could again connote that what is "caused" might be "cured."

As Doctors A. Elfin Moses and Robert O. Hawkins, Jr. remark
in their particularly detailed treatment on specific counseling: "lesbianism and homosexuality cannot be said to have an etiology" any
more than does heterosexuality. They advise that: "The helping
professional must be able to accept homosexuality and lesbianism
as viable orientations within this culture if he or she is to be of any
significant help to a lesbian or a gay man."

THE RIGHT TO LOVE

The fact is, of course, that the only problem whose cause should
be addressed is the ubiquitous presumption of heterosexuality as a
given. The question is not "Why am I gay?" but rather why should
persons be prohibited from loving whoever they do in fact love, and
concurrently, why have the intensely limited people who believe in
such prohibitions been permitted to keep 10% of the freest country
in the world under house arrest for 200 years? The answer is that we
live in a patriarchy, where enforced gender hierarchy and fetishized
reproduction are the mechanisms of control. And as these premises
surface in light of evolving national consciousness, some of the
patristic threads have begun to unravel, among them, the omission
of one whole race and one whole gender from the country's Constitution.

Now a small minority which has put itself in control of a mighty,
worldwide, tax-exempt, televangelist empire, dislikes such advances as have transpired. Energized, as have been Crusaders,
witch burners, and Iranian car bombers by a conviction that God
directs their actions, these neo-theocrats have set out to "rechristianize" across the board, reversing all liberties secured in excess of
their dogma, and improving upon extant oppression (as of the gay

community) with heretofore unexplored restrictions. In this interest did a small, fanatic oligarchy manage to dictate Republican Party platform for the whole of the 1980s. The following chapters will discuss the phenomenon of this formidable and growing American theocracy.

CHAPTER 4

POLITICS

"God hates orientation!" proclaimed Suffolk County, New York's fundamentalist Christians in opposition to a 1988 bill extending the Human Rights Commission's protection to men and women of the gay community. At the final hearings, after legislative passage, busloads of fundamentalists arrived to upbraid the County Executive who had said he was "inclined to sign" the measure into law. Hundreds and hundreds of "Christians" planted themselves for several consecutive days in the tiny legislative auditorium. Because the order of presentation could not be anticipated, speakers would lose their places in the lineup by emerging for air, food, or drink. Consequently gays defending the bill were trapped, so to speak, with the "Christians" for sometimes as long as eleven hours. The theocrats (proponents of government by religion) would identify a gay and mob around, Bibles aloft, shrieking passages from Leviticus prescribing death to "men who lay with men." Some of the dialogues which there ensued bring into sharp relief the premises by which a government founded in freedom of (and from) religion can be construed as an agent of doctrinal enforcement.

GOD HATES ORIENTATION!

One fundamentalist marshalled a placard which read in enormous black letters "GOD HATES ORIENTATION," the term's presumably having been misconstrued as meaning "homosexuality." Apparently the text had been reconsidered, for in what looked like lipstick, "hates" was deleted and "condemns" squeezed into the space above. "God hates the sin but loves the sinner," intoned the bearer from a place of majestic self-assurance. It was a sentiment left over from the days of Anita Bryant's pathological rampage to remove civil rights from gay Floridians in 1977. "I love you,

Sandy; I'm praying for you, sister," added another in exquisite condescension. This author had incurred double wrath by having requested introduction of the rights bill, on behalf of the grassroots group EEGO (East End Gay Organization) and by having, along with gay strategist Rich Amato, helped organize supporters for the sessions.

"Civil rights in the United States are not dependent on conformity to your religious beliefs," explained a pro-rights clergywoman. "You're the Devil trying to keep *GOD* [it was deafening] from running *His* country," was the reply.

This sentiment reflects the "religious right's" deliberate, ongoing strategy to undermine U.S. church/state separation. As early as 1976, Reverend Jerry Falwell declared: "The idea of religion and politics don't mix was invented by the Devil to keep Christians from running their own country."

Since then, many televangelists have maintained a steady drumbeat of such disinformation. It is a recurring theme in religious broadcasts that the nation's "satanists" have misconstrued the Constitution's First Amendment. Some evangelists claim that the Constitution presumed a government by "Christians," and that the exclusive intent of church/state separation was to prohibit government interference with Christianity and leave "Christians" free to enact their dogma through central government. This distortion, when it proceeds from any but the least sophisticated of broadcasters, is patent and intentional deception. While religious backgrounds do inform various perspectives (political and otherwise), the First Amendment clearly and specifically forbids "establishment of religion" by the state. That the Suffolk fundamentalists' rationale proceeded from televangelism was somewhat disturbing. That the televangelists were frequent White House guests was downright appalling.

But the round-faced Reverend Falwell was as at home with Ronald Reagan as was his fanatic agenda to "rechristianize" the country. In fact, a man often described as the President's best friend, Senator Paul Laxalt (R-NV) was the original sponsor of the formidable Family Protection Act (S.1808 9/24/79), the explicit purpose of which was to impose specific religious values through governmental institutions. This bill, which enjoyed many subsequent Congressional incarnations in the Reagan '80s, mandated public school instruction in stereotyped gender roles and sought to solidify fundamentalists' parental tyranny by exempting corporal punishment from the domain of child abuse. This philosophy persevered in the 1988 Republican Platform: "the God-given rights of the family come before those of government. That separates us from liberal Democrats."

"FAMILY" POLITICS

The Family Protection Act sought also to cloister females through tax disincentives to married women's working outside the home. And the bill restricted divorce, contraception, abortion, and *discussion* of "homosexuality as an acceptable alternative lifestyle" through restrictions on the Legal Services Corporation and on other federal funding. As anti-Equal Rights Amendment opponent Phyllis Schlafly explained in 1981: "If people decide not to have children . . . they should be forced to sign a piece of paper saying they will forfeit Social Security benefits."

While the Family Protection Act per se never flew, the agenda was not relinquished and the Administration persisted in implementing the various policies through regulative channels. Fragments of this bill emerged as a rule denying Federal funds to clinics *mentioning* abortion and a proposed "squeal law," withdrawn in a maelstrom of ridicule, to restrict minors' access to contraception. The "tuition tax credit" campaign is also a relic of the "family" colossus. Here the religionists, being unable to foment legislators sufficiently in the direction of state-subsidized catechism, wish to receive rebates for sending their children to indoctrinational "Bible schools," some of whose organizing principles actually include a "scripturally ordained" racial segregation.

THEOCRACY

It is odd that such conflation of religion and government got hold of what appeared to be the most worldly of administrations, the movie star's. The country had feared theocracy in John Kennedy, her first Catholic president. And on the campaign trail, JFK had taken pains to espouse U.S. separation of church and state. But, in the interest of "conservative" support, the 1980s Republicans simply ignored such trifles and actually wrote into the party platforms a personhood for the "unborn" belief, an anti-abortion judiciary appointment format, and an explicit Judeo-Christian bias which sorely tries the Constitution's Article VI forbidding any "religious test" from ever being "required as a qualification to any office or public trust under the United States."

Thus the religionists began dictating sectarian beliefs to the country's politicians. The "conservatives" turned out to be not conservative at all, but on the contrary, precipitously radical. They are, in fact, contemporary sun gods who issue "Christian" report cards rating candidates on issues as diverse as birth control and China policy. And the staunchest of traditional conservatives disavows them with intensity. After a spate of Congressional "court-stripping" attempts to remove the "moral" agenda from a judicial scrutiny it could not survive, the ordained "conscience" of the conservatives, Barry Goldwater (R-AZ) raved that he'd had a "stomachful" of social issues. "I don't think anyone on this floor wants another fight, especially over abortion. My wife founded Planned Parenthood in Arizona and she's been beating me to death on the subject" (*New York Times* 3/12/82).

Yet the fundamentalists, armed with the slickest computerized direct mail outfit in the country and a multibillion dollar international television empire, dictated, throughout the '80s, "traditional family/right-to-life" Republican platforms. The computer banks could trigger millions of threatening letters to media and Congress through vicious fundraising letters proclaiming, as did a mailing of August 13, 1981 that because "homosexuals do not reproduce" they "recruit" and are "out after my children and your children" signed: "In Christ, Jerry Falwell."

THE TAX-EXEMPT LOBBY

Although the tax-exempt status most ministries enjoy theoretically limits lobbying and partisan involvement, many televangelists became political oracles, maligning, across the board, candidacy for Jews, Muslims, atheists, and anyone not numbered among the "born-again" Christians. As one jolly son-of-a-senator turned evangelist so succinctly put it in the televised 1981 infancy of his eventual 1988 presidential primary: "The Constitution of the

United States, for instance, is a marvelous document for self-government by Christian people. But," bubbled Reverend Pat Robertson, "the minute you turn the document into the hands of non-Christian people and atheistic people they can use it to destroy the very foundation of our society." And, of course, these tax-exempt ministries recruit legions for their formally political appendages. Even as Falwell, just one solitary tentacle of this theopolitical gargantua, disbanded his fundraising/lobbying arm "Moral Majority," he projected his ministry's 1989 revenue at $140 million, up from the $88 million slump occasioned by an association with Jim and Tammy Baker's PTL (*New York Times* 6/12/89).

The fundamentalist agenda is a response to the mid-20th century's tentative release of "consensual adult privacy" from the jaws of "anti-pornographic" legislation. A major landmark in this progression was the Supreme Court's 1965 Griswold decision permitting the dissemination of birth-control wherewithal. In the dawning notion of privacy rights, FBI surveillance of gays relaxed, and the Post Office left off its practice of entrapping gays through the mail and tracing social contacts for purposes of alerting employers. Then, with the Kinsey and Hooker revelations about the ubiquity and normalcy of same-gender love (now printable, in the Court's growing understanding of such materials as not obscene) the massive lesbian/gay-male iceberg's tip emerged as a visible, viable, and considerable United States minority. These developments, in the '60s and '70s, triggered among fundamentalists a renewed conviction that the biblical literalism they consider normative should be imposed on everyone in the country. And while their effect has been especially pernicious for women and gay or minority men, the very concept of democracy has been, and continues to be, soundly trashed in a relentless and ongoing anti-intellectual crusade.

GOD'S CURRICULUM

One "Christian" battleground is the schools. Education being governmentally supervised, the U.S.A.'s public schools represent her "state." And an often articulated fundamentalist intent is to expressly "christianize" the public schools. This project, among many other things, includes the facilitation of organized school prayer, the prohibition of sex education, and an exhaustive manipulation of curricula through the removal and rewriting of educational materials, including the classics. To this end do the religionists participate in school board and state textbook selection, maintaining an onslaught on education that many had presumed neutralized by the 1925 Scopes trial.

Indeed, Tennessee's ridiculed anti-Darwinians and their stentorian champion, William Jennings Bryan, had been exquisitely dramatized in "Inherit the Wind," a much celebrated 1955 play by Robert E. Lee and Jerome Lawrence. But William Jennings Bryan *won* the Scopes trial, and the "monkey law" (forbidding the teaching of evolution) *stayed on* the books. Eventually "monkey laws" were replaced with "balanced treatment" policies whereby evolution could be mentioned but only if "creationism," the idea that God created the world six thousand years ago in six days, were also taught *as science* in the public schools.

Balanced Treatment

Although the U.S. Supreme Court's 1987 Edwards v. Aguillard decision prohibited state-*required* "balanced treatment," "creationism" can be and still is taught in the schools of some states. Meanwhile, textbook publishers, wishing representative books of which one edition will service the entire nation, either waffle around or completely avoid the major organizing principle of evolution. The result then, in the alternating ascendence of religion versus science, is an intermittent educational blackout concerning the emergence of biological species from previous primitive forms.

Contemporary "creation science" advocates argue that radiocarbon dating is invalid because "God could make old-looking rocks." They sometimes (as was related by Oberlin College biology professor, Michael Zimmerman) formally document themselves with citings from the *National Enquirer*. The title of Zimmerman's column in the April 14, 1987 Cleveland *Plain Dealer* summed it up well: "If it had merit, creationism would stand on it."

The authors of "balanced treatment" policies, including legislators and school boards, are presumably unable to understand that, while evolution is (like relativity) a theoretical explanation of extant data, its juxtaposition in education with an irrefutable mythology that contradicts such data invalidates all science from astrophysics to zoology. And it gets better. In 1987 the Arizona Governor's chief education aide testified on religious grounds against refutation of the flat earth theory.

Book Bannings

As for the more simplistic process of book banning per se, a virtual field day projects itself, perhaps into the 21st century. As reported by the civil liberties watchdog organization People For The American Way, the 1987-1988 school season saw 157 separate censorship incidents prohibiting sometimes whole anthologies. While contemporary authors John Steinbeck and Judy Blume enjoyed positions as the season's most frequently attacked authors, banishments also included Aristophanes' *Lysistrata* (circa 400 BCE) which promoted "women's lib" and Chaucer's *Canterbury Tales*.

The National Coalition Against Censorship, a New York-based clearinghouse, reports in regular bulletins that condemned works are often by or about people of color, including Gorden Parks' world famous novel *The Learning Tree* and Alex Haley's epic history *Roots*. Recent targets were *The Diary of Anne Frank* (some fundamentalists insist that the Nazi holocaust did not occur) and the *Merriam-Webster Collegiate Dictionary*. Sex education materials are routinely replaced with injunctions to celibacy. In Hawkins County Tennessee, the entire Holt Rinehart & Winston basic reading series was challenged on grounds that boys cooked, Macbeth's witches promoted the practice of magic, and Goldilocks wasn't punished for breaking into the three bears' house and stealing the porridge.

HOLDING THE LINE

The Supreme Court's 1982 Island Trees decision, limiting school boards' prescription of orthodoxy through book banning, has provided ground for education and library advocates. But the erosion of materials through fundamentalist narrowing of book selection continues. The 1988-89 season saw 172 separate censorship campaigns in 42 of the 50 states (New York *Daily News* 8/31/89). And a federally financed study conducted by the State University of New

York confirmed a profound curricular paucity in works by women and minority men (*New York Times* 6/21/89).

Any court tendency to hold the First Amendment line is being continually undermined by a judiciary appointment strategy, formally reaffirmed in the 1988 Republican Platform, which commits the Administration to screen judges for "traditional family values" as well as the "sanctity of innocent human life" anti-privacy rights philosophy. By the time Reagan left office, half the federal judgeships in the country had been selected in this vein. Two percent were Black and eight percent women. The litmus was Attorney General Edwin Meese's anti-abortion test, but church-state separation itself, and the gamut of "social" issues also hung in the very delicate balance.

In the last year of President Reagan's Administration, his three Supreme Court appointees, along with Byron White and Chief Justice William Rehnquist, retreated from decades of civil rights precedent in faithful execution of the Reagan Justice Department's agenda. And Congress' 1988 Civil Rights Restoration Act (to recoup earlier Court casualties) was passed *over a Reagan veto*. The next year, President Bush vetoed several measures authorizing government financed abortions for poor victims of rape and incest. As he explained to a group of horrified Republican Congresswomen, his specific intent was to obstruct any women desperate enough to allege rape in flight of their unintended pregnancies. Bush's first five judicial nominations were previously proposed by Ronald Reagan, and appointments continued in faithful obeisance to the fringe right.

BORK AND THE BALANCE

This was the "balance tipped" about which civil libertarians had been prophesying throughout the decade. With what condescension the U.S. electorate regarded the Republicans' anti-choice judiciary platforms as so many crumbs thrown to the "born-agains." How confident was mainstream U.S.A. that backward motion in civil rights was unthinkable; as confident as they were in losing the "monkey trial" that ridicule would disempower the anti-evolutionists. How odd that the threat went unrecognized until the judicial score was 4 to 4 with a vacancy in the swing seat. Then the prospect of 1987 Supreme Court appointee Robert Bork's blindness to privacy and desegregation took on a meaning his recently confirmed predecessor's (Antonin Scalia) practically identical mind-set had failed to inspire.

Of course, when the awakening coalition revitalized the women's movement with a massive 1989 march, half a million strong, for abortion choice, conservatives went on about "politicizing" the Court. But the real politicization was the Republicans' declared judiciary appointment format to effect through Court packing the host of policies toward which the Administration was unable to persuade Congress.

HARDWICK

In 1986 the Supreme Court simply savaged the Constitutional privacy premise underlying birth control and abortion rights in the Bowers v. Hardwick atrocity. Here, a margin of one arrested half a century's expansion of individual liberties to refuse same-gender relationships the privacy afforded non-gays. Tom Stoddard, Executive Director of the country's oldest gay legal advocacy organization, Lambda Legal Defense and Education Fund, called it the "Dred Scott case of the gay rights movement," a reference to the Court's 1857 refusal to recognize Blacks as citizens (*San Diego Union* 7/1/86).

The bitterly divided Court, which upheld a Georgia "sodomy" law, endorsed with its decision a police-state power to tell 10% of United States citizens with whom they could and could not make love. But, as the American Psychological Association and American Public Health Association had explained to the Court, those sexual practices Georgia defines as "sodomy," even though they are trotted out almost exclusively to harass and entrap gay people, are extremely common heterosexually. And the ruling now officially stigmatizes a considerable body of Americans with disabilities, in that for many such persons there are physically no alternatives to "sodomy."

The Hardwick decision did disavow "judgment on whether laws against sodomy between consenting adults in general, or between homosexuals in particular, are wise or desirable," implying that the road to gay citizens' privacy lay in repealing those "sodomy laws" the Court had just upheld. But although progress along these lines is being effected through some state courts, various species of "sodomy law" remain on the books in about half the country's states.

PRIVACY RIGHTS

The implications of Bowers v. Hardwick are as insidious as they are inflammatory. Although the police presence in the bedroom which occasioned Hardwick's arrest is relatively uncommon, the aura of "criminality" these archaic laws impart to the men and women of the gay community forms the basis for discrimination in all other areas. And, of course, in its rationale for this blatantly phobic decision, the Court exhumed the old reproductive schtick, proclaiming: "No connection between family, marriage or procreation on the one hand and homosexual activity on the other has been demonstrated."

Constitutionally protected privacy rights, such as they are, have been interpreted in several passages and through the Ninth Amendment's specification that "The enumeration in the Constitution, of certain rights, shall not be construed to deny or disparage others retained by the people." Privacy protections are afforded in some state constitutions. And specifics could, theoretically, be articulated in a Constitutional Amendment insulating "privacy" against the whims of a "conservative" Congress or an ideologically packed Court. In the immediate wake of the Hardwick decision, this author prepared a draft of such protection under the auspices of EEGO and with advice from Arthur Leonard of the Bar Association for Human Rights of Greater New York:

> The right to privacy in matters of birth control, abortion, and consensual sexual relations conducted in private shall not be abridged by the United States or by any State. (*"Consensuality" implies adulthood, perhaps tied to the Twenty-sixth Amendment's bestowal of voting rights at 18 years.*)

Although the concept has important cohesive and educational possibilities, the 1982 failure of the Equal Rights Amendment (ERA) has pointed up the difficulties involved in effecting the two-thirds Congressional and three-fourths state approval amendment passage requires.

A GAME PLAN

Current efforts seek to extend existing civil rights protections for housing, employment and public accommodation to groups distinguished by "affectional or sexual orientation." The ongoing national centerpiece is a comprehensive lesbian and gay civil rights bill, originally introduced in 1975 by Representative Bella Abzug (D-NY), and reintroduced in the 102nd Congress as the Civil Rights Amendments Act of 1991. Organizations such as Human Rights Campaign Fund, the impressive gay advocacy group and political action committee, often back candidates solely in proportion to their support for this measure. Also, many state, town, and county bills proceed along these lines. Of course such measures demand persistence. Massachusetts, Wisconsin, Hawaii, and Connecticut all protect gays. But the Connecticut bill took 18 years, and New York City's gay civil rights protection was 15 years in the making.

On the local level, measures can be initiated by a few citizens' talking to a bipartisan sample of their town boards. In East Hampton, New York, this author and another EEGO officer, Marie Manion, included the request for a resolution urging gay-positive County legislation in the successful campaign for a Town bill. Debra Lobel, a former Town Attorney, joined in the presentation. Local awareness is greatly facilitated when supplicants are "out," as was the case with all of the above. It is difficult for elected officials to oppose protection for persons they know

In the above case, a Town Board member, Tony Bullock (D), was eventually elected to the County legislature. This placed him in a position to introduce the controversial Suffolk County bill. For support, progressive allies were contacted. Regional Black civil rights groups and an independent-living organization for people with disabilities were regulars on the exhausting lobbying schedule. Both the East Hampton Town Supervisor, Judith Hope (D), and the Town Police Chief, Thomas Scott, wrote the County in support of gay legislation. A locally-based Republican legislator, Fred Thiele, bucked his party's hierarchy (to vote for the bill) and was re-elected with a record-breaking 75% of the vote. The National Organization for Women (NOW) chapters were enthusiastically on board with a strong lesbian/gay civil rights commitment. And several mainstream Protestant and Jewish groups were unequivocally supportive.

BIAS CRIME

Another vital rights area is the local, state and national campaign to curb a staggering increase in bias related violence. A 1987 study commissioned by the U.S. Justice Department (contract #OJP-86-002 10/7/87) shows that "Homosexuals are probably the most frequent victims" of such crimes. Gays of color are even more susceptible to violence than are whites; and the National Gay & Lesbian Task Force (NGLTF), a major lobbying and public education organization, cataloged for 1988, 7,248 incidents of anti-gay violence, many committed by right wing groups, including the Ku Klux Klan and the neo-Nazis (*New York Times* 6/8/89).

These crimes are sometimes impelled by the very authorities entrusted with their prevention. A Dallas judge actually reduced a murderer's sentence *because* the victims were gay: "I put prostitutes and gays at about the same level," said Jack Hampton of the State District Court, "and I'd be hard put to give somebody life for killing a prostitute" (*New York Times* 12/17/88). The next year a county district attorney in New York opposed the inclusion of "queers" in anti-violence protection because they are "sick people" (*New York Times* 3/6/89).

However, the very first gay-positive federal legislative enactment emerged on the bias crime frontier. In 1990 President Bush signed into law the Hate Crimes Statistics Act, commissioning the Justice Department to report crimes motivated by race, religion, ethnicity, or sexual orientation. This historic bill, of bipartisan Congressional sponsorship, was heavily lobbied by grassroots activists and will have wide reaching impact. Perhaps more such gay-inclusive language would result in fewer bias crimes to report.

SPECIAL PRIVILEGES

Another persistent prejudice is to the effect that civil rights for gays imply "special privileges." But existing civil rights codes explicitly enumerate protected minorities. And when the group most at risk is omitted, *that omission itself constitutes bias and occasions violence*. Also, figures regarding anti-gay violence fall dramatically short of the truth. Victims who may, through publicity, lose housing and employment are profoundly reluctant to report bias crimes. It is estimated that in New York City 80 to 90% of gay-bashings are undisclosed.

And a critical upswing in violence toward gays and people perceived as gay has been excited by the merciless stigmatization of gay males for their high AIDS incidence. The attendant fundamentalist rhetoric about God's retribution on gay men exacerbates widespread ignorance which seriously undermines the self respect essential to responsible relations within the community. Concurrently, the insidious Catholic hierarchy stifles AIDS education, enjoining heterosexuals to celibacy outside of marriage and lesbians and gay men to celibacy for life. Bishops' statements explicitly reject the use of condoms in AIDS prevention, recommending that homosexuals "form stable, chaste relationships" (*New York Times* 10/13/89). In other words, the Catholic Church would, through official opposition to established virus barriers, impose upon gay men under penalty of death, the sentence of lifelong celibacy to which it has been spectacularly unable to hold its own clergy, many of whom are also gay.

ON OUR OWN

Meanwhile it was the gay community per se that educated itself to the safer sex practices which are levelling off the rate of new infection in gay men and could, if the fanatics permit, save legions of non-gay people. As was remarked at the 1989 Montreal Conference by the Paris Pasteur Institute's Dr. Luc Montagnier, a discoverer of the virus (now called HIV) believed to cause AIDS, "many patients . . . are as well informed about AIDS as their doctors" (*New York Times* 6/13/89).

The outlook, however, is not great on the official educational front. Senator Jesse Helms (R-NC), through measures his colleagues often lack the courage to withstand, has seriously restricted the country's HIV disease information policies, finding clear explanations "pornographic" and refusing funds to educational groups who present gay relations in a positive or respectful light. Consequently, already rights-disadvantaged AIDS groups experience as genocide the government's coy resistance to explicit education. Meanwhile, women (particularly women of color) are being infected in increasing numbers. And in 1989, while the gay community spent valuable resources to effect the utterly obvious necessity for free speech regarding the pandemic, Blacks and Hispanics emerged with a staggering 42% of the nation's AIDS cases. On the up side, however, the vitriol of the opposition and the seriousness of the epidemic has made acceptable a degree of rights participation formerly considered too risky by some gays and sympathizers.

HIV AND CIVIL LIBERTIES

The AIDS front also involves a fight for the anti-discrimination measures and confidentiality which are so essential to medical treatment. A great many public health authorities have warned that fears of mandatory tests and exposure discourage concerned persons from voluntarily seeking either diagnoses or treatment. Yet "conservatives" continue to foment for coercive policies and even quarantine. In 1987, over the express objections of the Reagan Justice Department, the Supreme Court specifically held that people with contagious diseases were protected from unjustified discrimination by employers receiving federal funds. The ruling reflected the AMA's position that exclusionary policies must be based on medical evidence and not the "fear of contagion whether reasonable or not" for which basis the Administration had argued. Now rights advocates endeavor to extend the rationale of this decision to other areas of disability, including all phases of HIV-related discrimination. Of course, HIV is spread through blood transfusion (medical-procedure transmission is extremely rare), the sharing of hypodermic needles, and sexual practices which permit the exchange of blood, semen, or vaginal fluid. Such activities certainly constitute no recognized workplace or classroom occurrence.

Constant lobbying and judicial efforts proceed in the interest of funding and health care assistance. Daily battles rage with insurers who screen out "single males without dependents" and who endeavor to avoid payment of AIDS costs for established clients. On into the 1990s, HIV-infected U.S. citizens have continued to press for the facilitation of more drug testing and greater access to experimental products.

TREATMENT

A 1988 Food and Drug Administration policy permitting the country's doctors to import unapproved drugs for the terminally ill was something of a boon. For throughout the '80s, with first no antivirals and later only one exorbitant product approved, U.S. residents routinely pilgrimaged to France and other nations in search of foreign prescriptions for medications not even being considered in the States. Then in 1989 the director of the National Institute of Allergy and Infectious Diseases called for "parallel track" access to unapproved but potentially useful drugs of established safety. One result was a legal, if expensive "buyers club" to import European and Mexican medicines.

But many such advances as have been made are the result of incessant prodding by health advocates like the Washington, DC-based AIDS Action Council and National Association of People With AIDS, or from community activists like ACT-UP (AIDS Coalition to Unleash Power), whose dramatic street theater few can ignore. AIDS efforts have generally proceeded in a governmental context ranging anywhere from hostility to oblivion. The September 2, 1989 *New York Times* reported that Reagan's own physician said the President did not grasp the seriousness of HIV infection until Rock Hudson became ill in 1985, years after the disease had been identified. "He accepted it like it was measles and it would go away," said Brigadier General John Hutton, MD.

THE MILITARY FRONT

In recent years, gay rights issues have covered a panorama of U.S. life, including an important move, successful in 1990, to reverse the immigration law's exclusion of lesbians and gay men. On the military front, reversal is sought for the bigoted Pentagon policy which proclaims homosexuality incompatible with military service and which has kept the country's gay and lesbian soldiers perhaps more closeted than any other single group. But retired service people participate yearly as Gay Veterans in Pride Day parades, much to the apoplectic chagrin of homophobic groups. And in 1989 it developed that a comprehensive interdisciplinary analysis, released only after months of pressure from rights advocates, had been commissioned by the Defense Department itself. The study, "Nonconforming Sexual Orientations and Military Suitability" (PERS-TR-89-002 12/88), along with a less formal work in its wake, showed no relationship between sexual orientation and military performance or security risk, and recommended that the military reconsider its exclusionary policy.

Citing statistics showing civilian gay men and lesbians *were at least as likely as heterosexuals* to have military histories, the researchers, Theodore R. Sarbin, PhD, and Kenneth E. Karols, MD, PhD, explained that by "reasonable assumption" numbers "as high as 10 percent" of military personnel *are* lesbians and gay men who complete their service undetected. A fracas of memos was also exhumed, with officials castigating researchers who would impugn military policy and berating the research agency for permitting such work to proceed. The experts in the Defense Department study group explained, as do biologists to creationists, that research whose conclusion is foregone is not research at all (*Washington Post* 11/6/89).

The reports were formally rejected for "exceeding" their mandate, and their very existence was denied until a cover page surfaced during Lambda Staff Attorney Sandra Lowe's investigation of one of the 10,000 gay related military separations which have occurred since 1982. Eventually, Congressional pressure from Representatives Gerry Studds (D-MA) and Patricia Schroeder (D-CO) induced a "leak" of the studies. These new gay "Pentagon Papers" are extremely significant. Drawing an apt comparison with "the same kind of discrimination that Blacks and women faced" when they originally sought to serve, Lowe observed: "it is now patently obvious that the military's policy of discrimination is the product of prejudice, pure and simple" (Lambda press release 10/24/89).

Watkins

A significant 1989 federal appeals court ruling required the Army to re-enlist former Staff Sergeant Perry Watkins on grounds that he was, with the Army's full knowledge of his orientation, repeatedly re-enlisted throughout his exemplary 14-year career. The American Civil Liberties Union had represented Watkins since 1981, when Army regulations tightened to exclude the homosexually oriented as well as the homosexually active. Attorney Nan Hunter, as Director of the ACLU's Lesbian and Gay Rights Project, called the ruling's characterization of Watkins as respected by his peers and of great benefit to the Army "a total repudiation of the rationale for the Army's exclusionary policy" (*Gay Community News* 5/14/89). But this decision confined itself to the specifics of Watkins' case, side-stepping the larger issue of whether the blanket exclusion of lesbian and gay Americans violates the Constitution's guarantee of "equal protection." And the Bush Administration sought review of even this narrow ruling, which, nonetheless the Supreme Court did let stand in 1990. The issue is further complicated by limits on court authority in military matters. Now activists are pushing for a Congressional move to reverse the exclusionary policy per se. Meanwhile, massive military witch hunts persist with considerably higher discharge percentages among lesbians than gay men.

DOMESTIC BENEFITS

That "family" has become code for state enforced anti-gay policies motivates an interest in the recognition of a "family diversity" among those whom the government formally forbids the nicety of legal relationship. In this vein, "alternate families" claim some of the host of privileges marriage conveys vis-à-vis pensions, taxation, insurance options, survivorship, and hospital visitation. This move-

ment achieved a major presence in 1989 when the San Francisco
Board of Supervisors unanimously passed legislation permitting
lesbian, gay and unmarried heterosexual couples to register "domestic partnerships" defined as "two people who have chosen to
share one another's lives in an intimate and committed relationship." Several U.S. cities provide similar protection, but the San
Francisco measure was later defeated in a public referendum orchestrated by the Roman Catholic Church. Comparable enactments
will be attempted in Boston and also in New York, where the
State's highest court has recognized same-gender relationships in
the context of rent-control tenancy survivorship. And across the
country, labor unions continue to negotiate health insurance and
bereavement leave benefits for city employees in self-defined kin-
ships.

SHARON KOWALSKI

Dramatic inequities are wrought by the religiously based exclusion of gays from the legal protections of marriage. The injustice
was brought sharply into focus by the outrageous situation of
Sharon Kowalski, an adult who sustained serious brain injuries in a
1983 accident. Shortly after the accident, Kowalski's father obtained exclusive legal guardianship and isolated Sharon from her
life partner, Karen Thompson, a university professor who was providing daily physical and occupational therapy for Kowalski. After
three and one half years of court battles, medical re-evaluation,
resisted by Kowalski's father, indicated in 1989 that Sharon should
be receiving extensive therapy not available at the nursing home
where her father had her imprisoned. In 1989 Thompson's lawyer
persuaded a judge that Kowalski could in fact interact with others
(she used mechanical word-selection devices) and the couple were
permitted visitation. Kowalski had made it very clear that she considered Thompson her lover. However, Thompson was still not
granted guardianship and Sharon's father, who refused to acknowledge his daughter as a lesbian, insisted he did "not believe the
reports that she was happy to see Thompson" (*New York Times* 2/8/
89).
    Of course, the biological families of lesbians and gay men are

also at risk. Gay parents sometimes lose custody of their children to less suitable heterosexual ex-spouses. Adoption policies often screen out gays. However, a growing body of evidence is now proving that lesbian or gay male environments are in no way deleterious to children and that families do not influence orientation. These revelations are beginning to facilitate some legal victories for gay parents. Also now, increasing numbers of lesbian couples are conceiving through artificial insemination. One San Francisco-based organization, the National Center For Lesbian Rights, maintains a strong focus on such areas of family law, particularly vis-à-vis lesbians of color.

MEANWHILE, BACK AT THE HEARINGS . . .

Suffolk's rights bill was, in fact, eventually signed into law. But not before the fundamentalists raved repetitively from the works of a militaristic and graphically violent poet. This attempt to discredit gays was roughly equivalent to defaming heterosexuals because the Marquis de Sade was one. And the fundamentalists brought with them their very young children, exposing those whom they purported to "protect" to material none of the attending gay and lesbian professionals, teachers, attorneys, or physicians considered remotely suitable for minors. Red-faced, a "minister," complete with clerical collar, waved an AIDS education pamphlet accusing: "this book teaches our children to have anal [it rhymed with panel] sex." Dolores Klaich, author of the lesbian chronicle classic *Woman Plus Woman*, rose to explain that the intent of AIDS education was not salacious. In the lobby a fundamentalist hissed that "they" wanted to sell "condos" (he meant condoms) in the school washrooms. One woman, Dr. Rose Walton, was booed when she described herself as a "lesbian and a Christian." A seasoned speaker, she manifested visible tears by the end of her cogent report on HIV disease. The malice in the room was a physical weight.

This author remarked that Jesus had said nothing about homosexuality and pandemonium ensued. "Read the Gospels" shouted the fundamentalists. "There is nothing about gays in the Gospels," I raved wildly to the audience. "Please address your remarks to the chair, Ms. Rapp," reprimanded County Executive Patrick Halpin.

Irene Gould, a septuagenarian refugee of Nazi Germany, characterized the climate as "early Third Reich." Later that day, when Long
Island's most sophisticated gay lobbyist, Rich Amato, addressed
the group about escalating violence against the community, his
voice broke like a teenaged boy's.

The Suffolk fundamentalists, in unwavering commitment to the
destruction of their own democracy, enjoyed several subsequent
days of sermonizing in two of what proved to be unsuccessful recall
attempts. The rights bill, which simply expanded the domain of an
investigative commission, was eventually signed by the valiant
County Executive. Some of the gays lost their jobs for appearing.

EDUCATION

Many non-fundamentalists, elected representatives among them,
do share the premises brought into such sharp relief by the Suffolk
action. Some, who would be horrified to number themselves among
the fanatics, cling to a suspicion that gay orientation should weaken
a person's civil rights. It is these persons who are amenable to education with respect to psychological realities. For such educational
purposes, national figures have provided statements from which
rights defenses can be prepared.

Dr. Calderone

For example, the bizarre but persistent notion that equal rights
will occasion a "contagion" of same-gender orientation from
school teachers to their students can be countered with the testimony of Mary S. Calderone, MD, of the Sex Information and Education Council of the U.S. (SIECUS): "no one can *choose* to be
either heterosexual or homosexual, neither of which states depends
upon sexual acts but is specifically a state of being. Furthermore, no
one who was programmed by five years of age to be heterosexual
can be seduced to become homosexual, any more than the reverse."

Outrageously enough, some legislators seem possessed of the notion that lesbians and gay men could obtain equal rights by leaving
off loving their partners and undergoing brain-washing to induce

heterosexual behavior or celibacy. Those of this mind-set Calderone enjoins to ask any psychiatrist if "10 percent of our population could be 'cured' of its homosexuality. First we'd have to learn by what process we might 'cure' heterosexuality."

Dr. Marmor

Along the same lines, Judd Marmor, MD, past President of the American Psychiatric Association, explained in 1980 that: "People do not 'choose' to be homosexual any more than they 'choose' to be heterosexual. In almost all instances, the basic factors that lead to a homosexual propensity are established before the age of six, well before the school years even begin. . . . That modeling is not a relevant factor, in any event, is indicated by the fact that all homosexuals come from heterosexual families, and that the overwhelming majority of the 'models' they are exposed to in our culture are heterosexual."

The APA

In this vein did the American Psychological Association, representing over "70,000 members, including the vast majority of psychologists holding doctoral degrees from accredited universities in the United States," submit a brief of amicus curiae (No.85-4006 Ninth Circuit U.S. Court of Appeals 8/30/88) on behalf of Sergeant Perry Watkins in his contested separation from the United States Army (discussed above). They argue that gays deserve the Fourteenth Amendment's "equal protection" which is afforded to groups distinguished by immutable or largely involuntary characteristics. Citing first A. Damien Martin and Eli Coleman, then Gerald C. Davison and Alan K. Malyon (all doctors), the brief explains respectively that: "at a minimum, the majority of homosexuals are unable to change their sexual orientation, even if they were to wish to do so," and that "it is ethically questionable, from the point of view of a practitioner, to seek to alter through therapy a trait that is not a disorder and is extremely important to individual identity."

DUCKS

Such arguments may be brought to bear on rational people. But logic does not obtain for those who define faith as eschewing evidence. Repeated testimony to the effect that the overwhelming preponderance of sexual child abusers are heterosexual men did not dissuade Suffolk's fundamentalists from distributing flyers implying that the human rights bill promoted "child-molestation." Of course, these matters have to do with "age of consent" laws which are in no way addressed by such legislation. And at one point the anti-gays sent out a press release proclaiming that sex with animals had been legalized throughout Suffolk. One of the local papers ran a column about the immorality of sex between humans and ducks.

ETERNAL VIGILANCE

Suffolk's anti-gay legislators, a minority by dangerously narrow numbers, continually threaten the local community with the specter of another inflammatory recall vote. Meanwhile, on the national scene, lesbian/gay advocates had actually to defend the Department of Health and Human Services gay youth suicide findings (discussed in Chapter 1) from the Department itself: "We believe . . . that suicide and violence are not family values," wrote Urvashi Vaid, Executive Director of the National Gay & Lesbian Task Force. Through youths "destroying their lives, families are undermined rather than strengthened," she continued in a September 11, 1989 letter to President Bush.

It seems that Congressman William Dannemeyer (R-CA) had found the suicide statistics antithetical to "traditional family values" and wished parts of the report arbitrarily "denounced." He was particularly offended by a conclusion that the "root problem of gay youth suicide is a society that discriminates against and stigmatizes homosexuals while failing to recognize that a substantial number of its youth has a gay or lesbian orientation." He also objected to the report's explanation of homosexuality as "not a mental illness or disease" and confused the recognition of homosexually oriented youth with "homosexual recruitment" and "child-molestation." Then, in a bizarre "shoot the messenger" passage,

Congressman Dannemeyer called upon the Administration to "dismiss from public service all persons still employed" who had prepared the report (letter to President Bush 9/7/89).

What's more incredible is that Louis Sullivan, MD, the Bush Administration's Secretary of Health and Human Services, responded to Representative Dannemeyer's complaints by agreeing that the study's views ran contrary to his (Sullivan's) agenda for "advancing traditional family values." He declined to "approve" the report and further pledged to screen future initiatives to the end of their helping "to advance, first and foremost, the role of family, as well as that of faith" (letter to Dannemeyer 10/13/89).

SECTARIAN BELIEFS ARE NOT UNIVERSALS

With such sentiment now crystallized into a Hydra-headed political monster, the United States must leave off the tradition that it is "bad manners" to argue religion. Clearly, religionists are in place at the highest of elected and appointed office. At the very least, their theological premises must be exhumed and examined. If nothing else, the debate exposes these beliefs to be not the universals their proponents presume, but rather those very same narrow sectarian tenets whose establishment in government the U.S. Constitution strictly forbids.

Although psychology does not compute among many fundamentalists, religion does. As fire is often best fought with fire, so through a challenge to primary religious footings can a presumed divine right of men to the control of women and gays be countered. Many of the nation's theocrats are, as it happens, as short on theology as they are long on ardor. The following chapters will consider those theological developments and perspectives that dispute their philosophies. The discussion will begin with a look at how the theocratic incursion on U.S. privacy rights impacts upon heterosexuals through mandated reproduction.

Suffolk OKs Gay Rights Bill

Would Have Rights Unit Investigate Charges Of Discrimination; Halpin 'Inclined to Sign It'

Page 3

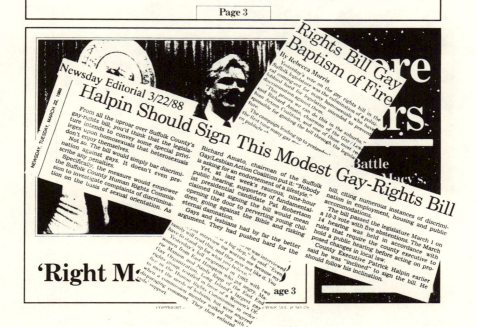

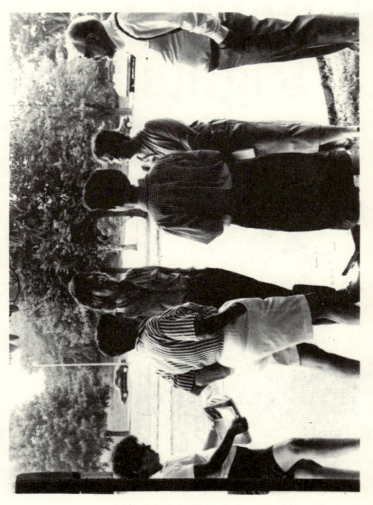

East Hampton Star interviews the author after passage of the East Hampton Town lesbian/gay rights measure 8/16/1985. Left to right with former affiliations: Vivian Shapiro—Human Rights Campaign Fund National Chair, Marie Manion—EEGO Co-chair, Sandy Rapp—EEGO Political Committee Co-chair, Joanne Furio—reporter conducting interview, Debra Lobel Atty., Bill Hirsch—EEGO Political Committee Co-chair. photo: Cal Norris (courtesy East Hampton Star)

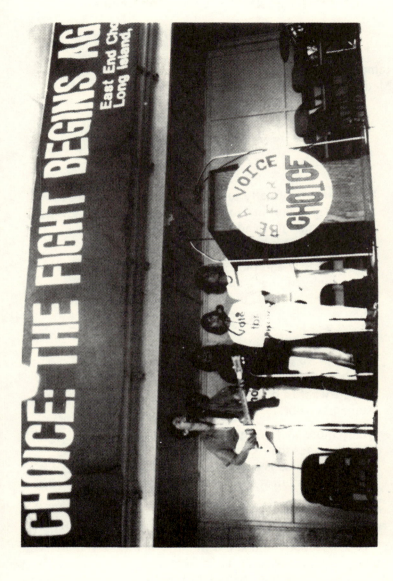

The author leads the East End Women's Alliance Singers in "Remember Rose: A Song for Choice" at a National Women's Day Rally in East Hampton, NY, 1989. Left to right are Sandy Rapp, Dolores Karl, Frances Alenikoff, Astrid Myers, Lea Abrams. photo: Jackson Friedman

REMEMBER ROSE: A Song for Choice

© Sandy Rapp 1989

"Remember Rose" is about the first casualty of the 1977
Medicaid-abortion cutoff. The story was documented
by Ellen Frankfort and Frances Kissling in

Rosie: The Investigation of a Wrongful Death
[Frankfort 79]

Rosie Jimenez finally turned up dead,
So the paper said in Texas.
Finally turned up dead, after Medicaid
Restrictions took her choice away.

Televangelists and their politics
Made Jenny Jimenez an orphan.
Praying in the light, bombing in the night,
They wave their roses red but Rose is dead.

chorus:
Get your laws off me; I'm not your property;
Don't plan my family, I'll plan my own.
I don't want to be in your theocracy;
Remember liberty, Remember Rose.

Many more will go by the way of Rose
And the ones that went before her.
Unless a course is set, present and direct,
Because "a chill wind blows" and Rose is dead.

[Rapp 89]

"Jenny" is a pseudonym taken from the book. "A chill wind
blows" was the phrase used by U.S. Supreme Court Justice Harry
A. Blackmun in his stirring dissent to the 1989 Webster decision
permitting an expansion of state restriction on abortion.

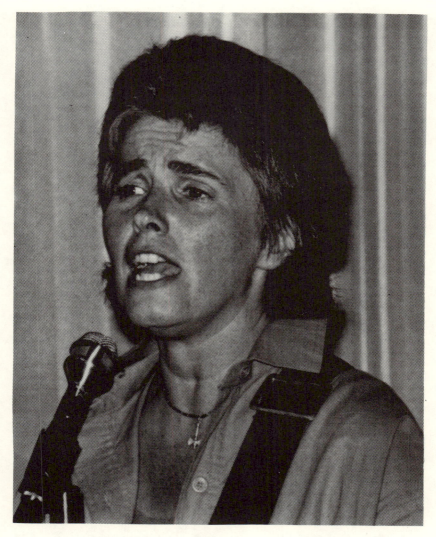

The author in concert at the Women's Coffee House in the Lesbian & Gay Community Services Center, NYC.
photo: © 1986 Morgan Gwenwald

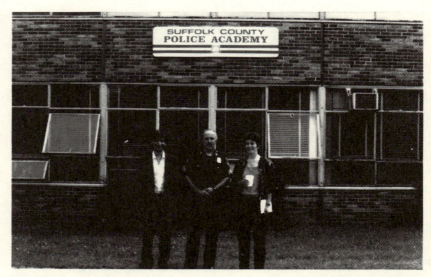

Gay Sensitivity Training is conducted by the author and gay activist Rich Amato, pictured above with Sergeant Tom Martorano and below with Detective Sergeant Joseph C. Zito, Commanding Officer of the Suffolk County Police Department's Bias Crimes Bureau.

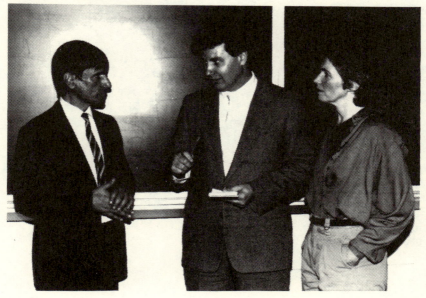

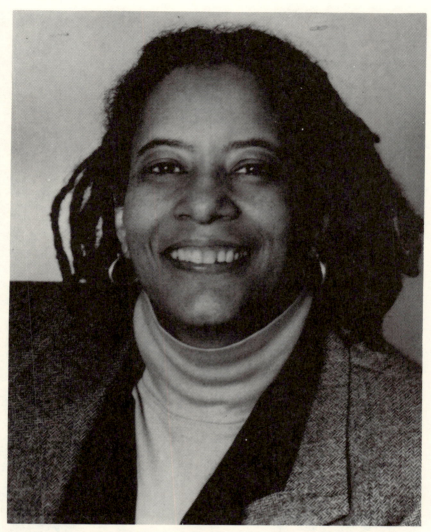

Sandra J. Lowe is a Lambda Legal Defense and Education Fund Staff Attorney. Lowe's investigation smoked out a 1988 Pentagon report showing that the Defense Department itself has found lesbians and gay men to be at least as well adjusted as their heterosexual counterparts.
photo: Tom Tyburski (courtesy LLDEF)

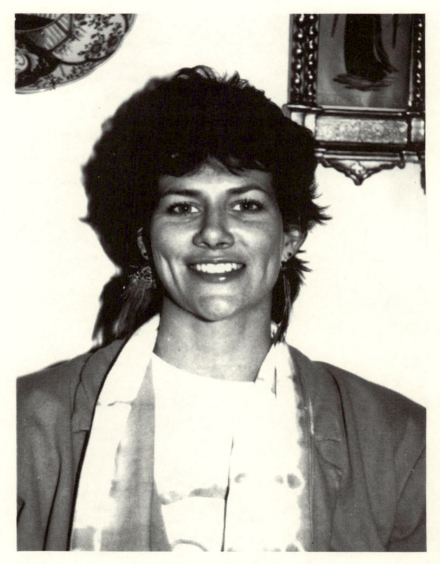

Nancy Karl is a psychic and AIDS care volunteer. Of contemporary anti-gay moralists she says: "the judgement acts as a spotlight on the *judges'* existences." photo: Mary Stedman Weinstock 1990

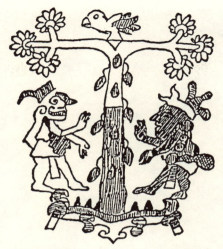

The Tau from a Maya Manuscript

The Tree of Life or "Tau" is a universal symbol which far antedates the Christian cross. (reproduction courtesy BE Books/Brotherhood of Life: Churchward 88)

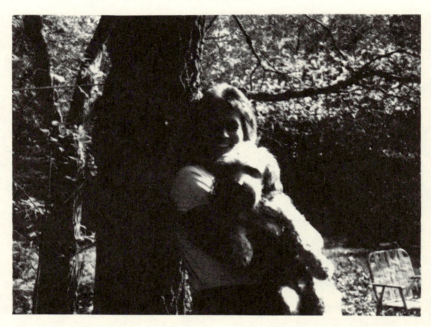

The author in her back yard with Cagney, a golden female terrier mix.
photo: Anne L. Butler

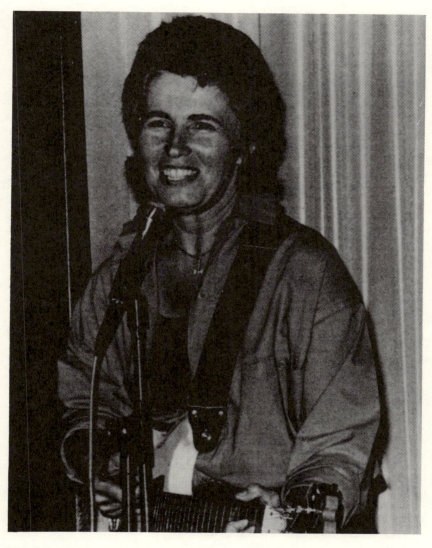

The author in concert at the Women's Coffee House in the Lesbian & Gay Community Services Center, NYC.
photo: © 1986 Morgan Gwenwald

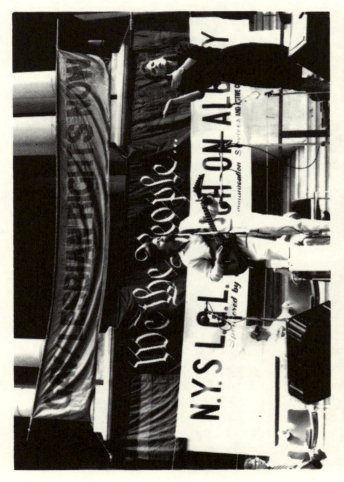

New York State Lesbian & Gay Lobby March on Albany in 1990. The author sings an original: "White Men In High Places," as Trudy Caldon, a professional interpreter, signs for the deaf. In the background (left to right) are Tim Mains, an openly gay Rochester City Councilman and Morris Kight, a legendary Los Angeles-based founder of the contemporary lesbian/gay liberation movement. The photo was taken by former New York Air National Guard Lieutenant Ellen Nesbitt, who is currently contesting a discharge based solely on sexual orientation.

CHAPTER 5

ABORTION

In 1984 the United States fundamentalists went global with a policy presented at the International Conference on Population in Mexico City. Through this travesty, the Reagan Administration simply defunded worldwide any organizations whose subgrantees or sub-subgrantees trafficked in *information* about pregnancy termination, even with one half of one percent of their non-U.S. funds. Among major casualties were the two most effective family planning institutions in the world: United Nations Population Fund (UNFPA), which devotes its resources to offsetting the inevitable doubling of the planet's population (now at over 5 billion) by 2025 (*Washington Post* 5/17/89), and International Planned Parenthood Federation (IPPF), whose constitution precludes its imposing pronatalism upon foreign affiliates.

THE MEXICO CITY POLICY

Through the Mexico City Policy, our U.S.A., the heretofore undisputed leader in population education, has become part of the problem it helped to define, exporting pronatalism in countries only recently induced to recognize the crisis of unchecked growth. In service of the policy, textbooks, which might have educated famine ridden populations about contraception, have been literally destroyed because the States would defund educators for possession [Camp 87].

In spite of the fact that, even under previously established policy, no U.S. funds in any way ever facilitated abortion, UNFPA was zapped for its efforts in China, where an incentive policy on abortion is officially non-coercive. Although local abuses are sometimes reported, the program itself is absolutely essential. It is in place for the purpose of averting another such famine as took the lives of as many as 30 million Chinese between 1958 and 1962 [ZPG 90].

To date, the most serious problems are in India (growing at 1.4 million per month) where some U.S. organizations report that they simply cannot function effectively, and in Latin America where U.S. Cooperating Agencies are unable to work with women's organizations because of the groups' advocacy for abortion choice. In other words, the United States is stifling free speech globally, taking with it much contraceptive research and sex education, thereby precipitating more, not fewer abortions. And a similar domestic "gag rule" was, in 1990, slated for Supreme Court review. This put the U.S. in a position of promulgating abroad restrictions whose constitutionality was seriously questioned within her own borders.

Ominously, the "Mexico City" effects will become even more widespread in times to come. Some long-term grantees are insulated until new grants redefine eligibility. Challenged but unchecked, the policy is a very bad joke, played tragically upon a global and perhaps cosmic stage. In 1988 The Club of Earth, a group of National Academy of Sciences members, described "overpopulation and rapid population growth" as "intimately connected" with the "depletion of non-renewable resources, deterioration of the environment and increasing international tensions." They declared that "arresting global population growth" was an issue which "should be second in importance on humanity's agenda only to avoiding nuclear war" (Long Island *Newsday* 9/4/88).

THE RETREAT FROM ROE

Meanwhile, the United States, adding a yearly 2 million to this incipient planetary ghetto, is fast catching up to her own exported moralism. In 1989 the Reagan Court began an earnest retreat from 1973's landmark Roe v. Wade decision establishing early abortion as a Fourteenth Amendment "liberty" of which persons may not be deprived. Roe permitted state regulation in the interest of women's health only after the first three months, its having been firmly established that modern legal abortion was much safer than childbirth in the first "trimester." Restriction on behalf of the fetus was prohibited until the third "trimester," its being the case that fetuses are not capable of survival outside the womb until about 24 weeks' gestation.

In spite of the fact that this "viability" mark is not expected to alter, even with improved technology, the Supreme Court's 1989 Webster v. Reproductive Health Services decision presumed a four-week margin of error to permit state requirement of expensive and intrusive viability determination tests in the 20th week. More frighteningly, a plurality of judges argued that state interest in a fetus might legitimately exist before viability, implying even possible first trimester incursion into what was described by Justice Harry Blackmun (author of Roe) in his unforgettable dissent to Webster as "the quintessentially intimate, personal and life-directing decision" around the right to which "millions of women and their families have ordered their lives."

BIRTH CONTROL AT RISK

Even more dramatically, the Court intimated an attack on *contraception* by failing to address a statute preamble equating personhood with egg fertilization, a theological premise under whose auspices "right-to-lifers" have for years been advocating the proscription of most birth control. Because many contraceptives, including the IUD and some pills, prevent uterine implantation of already fertilized eggs, anti-abortionists define them as abortifacients which "kill persons." Consequently, the U.S.A.'s research and market frontier, already badly intimidated by the country's penchant for product liability litigation, is a Reagan decade behind the safer and more effective advances now available elsewhere. The subcutaneous five-year hormone implant was a staple abroad years before its Food and Drug Administration (FDA) approval in late 1990. Other hostages held by religionists include injection contraceptives, external skin "badges," "morning-after" pill research, and of course RU 486, a safe, effective drug which the French use (in combination with a prostaglandin agent) to terminate early pregnancies inexpensively and without surgery.

Furthermore, Webster permitted an escalation in state restriction of funded abortions, including privately paid operations at public facilities. This phenomenon creates among women many of the delays and hence late abortions to which the religionists so loudly object. And any abortion funding restrictions, of course, result in dramatic tax expenditures. Women who would receive publicly funded abortions are also eligible for publicly funded childbirth, neonatal care, and often 18 years of child support.

JUSTICE O'CONNOR

In the pivotal Webster decision, Justice Sandra Day O'Connor was, it seems, the one to hold the rights line from even worse erosion. O'Connor ruminated ominously that another occasion would better serve to examine Roe "carefully." But she implied some respect for choice with a citing that "regulation imposed on a lawful abortion is not unconstitutional unless it unduly burdens the right to seek an abortion." The problem is that many dramatic obstacles seem not to strike O'Connor as "undue."

Of course, almost all regulation has burden at its intent. Fewer than 1% of abortions occur after the 20th week. And only one-tenth of one percent (.01%) are performed after viability, many of these with such compelling contingencies as a severely abnormal fetus, or a woman whose health is at grave risk (*Newsweek* 7/17/89). Over 90% of abortions are performed in the first trimester, and attempts to force cost-prohibitive hospital licensing standards on the efficient clinics which perform most U.S abortions are patently unnecessary for this simplest of surgical procedures. Of course, a combination of sonar tests and licensing requirements could, in the wink of a Justice's eye, effectively, if not literally, overrule Roe for most U.S.A. women by transforming the cost of an abortion from about $200 to about $2,000.

PARENTAL INVOLVEMENT

Also, Webster's incursion on Roe v. Wade poised the Court for its 1990 rulings to permit required parental notification for minors seeking abortions. These restrictions are, of course, extremely perilous, in that they force youth underground in cases where violence is expected from an estranged or hostile parent. One Indiana teenager, Becky Bell, died from a clandestine abortion in 1988 simply because she was unwilling to *disappoint* the parents who now campaign at a national media level against parental consent and notification laws.

Nor does "judicial bypass" of parental involvement resolve the problem. Many teenagers are at least as apprehensive of judges (numbers of whom are expressly anti-abortion) as they are of their own parents. And the "bypass" procedure itself invites dangerous and costly delays. It is also somewhat ludicrous to presume that a girl old enough to be pregnant is not old enough to know she does not want to be pregnant or, even worse, that consent laws should confer upon parents the right to impose childbirth when abortion is the safer alternative. Do parents then also enjoy the right to impose abortion?

MORE U.S. WOMEN DIE

Meanwhile, major women's groups wrestle the fundamentalist lobby to permit importation and manufacture of RU 486, a product which could remove the need for most surgical abortion, transforming clinics the religionists now storm into backup facilities for the drug's minute failure incidences. Other groups, in the ominous new atmosphere, are publishing manuals for early home suction abortion, which, *if* performed under sterile conditions, may provide some alternative to the filthy back street coat hanger of the recent past. But misused suction kits will wreak infection just as deadly as the scrapings of old. And legislatively, state battles will rage without end until a Congressional standard for abortion rights is established.

A Freedom of Choice Act could prohibit states from restricting pre-viability abortions. But absent a sea change in the Administration, a Presidential veto would be inevitable. Thus poor women, unable to travel to rights conscious states, will simply experience obstacles, complications, and death in greater numbers. Predictably, the economic tailoring will be most oppressive to minorities. The first documented casualty of the 1977 Medicaid abortion cutoff was Rosie Jimenez, a 27-year-old Mexican American student, mother to a young girl [Frankfort 79]. As was remarked by Byllye

Avery of the National Black Women's Health Project: "Racism is the time of day. It's no accident that the erosion of abortion rights is happening at the same time as racism's second coming . . . They are using the wombs of women to play political football" [RCAR 88].

JUDICIAL PHILOSOPHIES

Justice O'Connor's recurring references to the trimester framework as "problematic" seem to imply at least some recognition of pre-viability as occasioning abortion rights. Justice Scalia actually berated her for a perceived reluctance to overturn the Roe landmark, complaining that the public would continue to prevail upon him to "follow the popular will" despite the fact that judges were appointed for life in order to "follow the law despite the popular will." What he seems not to grasp is that he and his recent colleagues were appointed *because* of their non-discovery of unenumerated privacy rights in the country's Constitution, and that many citizens, presuming a United States Constitution by and for the people as defensive of their bodily integrity, look to the courts to protect them from, rather than enforce upon them, the tyranny of a handful of well-financed religious zealots.

Whether through elitism that precludes his recognizing any stab at Constitutional interpretation on the part of the "public," or through an idealism which truly does affect his reason, the politics Justice Antonin Scalia decries as inappropriate to the Court are precisely what put him there. Described almost universally as "brilliant," one may ask to what avail is brilliance in the service of religious tyranny. Scalia's dissent in Edwards v. Aguillard (1987), on what many libertarians would call the William Jennings Bryan side of the evolution question, was to the effect that, since the religious intent proceeded from the fundamentalists' "creation science" witnesses and not from the duped, scientifically naive Louisiana State Legislators, "balanced treatment" for biblically based creationism could become law of the land.

Justice Anthony Kennedy's immediate alignment with the most conservative members of the Court rendered the success of the anti-Bork campaign (which blocked Reagan's first choice for retiring Justice Lewis Powell's seat) somewhat short-lived. Only a declared pro-choice, pro-privacy rights philosophy could preclude a given nominee's subscription to the personhood for the "unborn" religious criterion affirmed in recent Republican platforms. But Kennedy, in Bork's wake, was confirmed by the Senate through scant judicial record and perhaps through civil libertarians' exhaustion. Justice Kennedy has shown no reluctance whatever to undermine the meticulous compromise Roe v. Wade delineated between women's autonomy and the states' "interest" in a fetus at "viability."

VIABILITY

This "viability" moment, on which the nation's attention is so riveted as the point at which a state may or may not seize its female citizens, does have historic precedent. Until 1800 abortion before "quickening" (the mid-gestation perceptibility of fetal movement) was permitted nationwide under the country's assumption of British common law.

Then the 19th century saw a criminalization move orchestrated by physicians eager to wrest reproductive domain from unorthodox competitors, among whom, of course, were numbered the midwives. The medical community, some of whom did concurrently express concern for developing life, advocated a purely reproductive role for women, opposed liberalized divorce laws, and fought the admission of women to its profession. Among reasons these doctors gave for this moral crusade was the tendency of Catholics to outbreed the U.S.-born, white Protestants so predominantly represented in their own ranks [Mohr 78].

A state by state campaign effectively criminalized abortion by the end of the century, but the only national policy touching on the subject was the 1873 Comstock Act which defined as pornography all printed matter on abortion and birth control. This phenomenon alone should convince feminists attracted to "anti-porn" legislation that civil rights are immensely more endangered by censorship than they are advanced.

The anti-abortion crusade in the United States was an attempt to consolidate reproductive domain under the confines of the newly formed American Medical Association. Further intent was in the interest of women, some of whom were being poisoned by the herbal abortifacients in use at the time. The early religious community was vastly uninterested in the abortion matter and the current "fetal rights" rhetoric is very much a last ditch strategy to avert an evolving women's consciousness from autonomy and self-determination.

ENSOULMENT

Even the Catholic Church, whose colossal financial subsidy launched the current anti-choice crusade, did not equate conception with personhood until the late 19th century. In fact, throughout much of Church history, predominant theologians, including Saint Augustine and Saint Thomas Aquinas, assumed "ensoulment" of a fetus occurred at 40 days in males and 80 in females. This "ensoulment" tenet presumes, in Aristotelian tradition, that the actualizing principle of personhood is separate from the fetal vehicle which is being formed. But "ensoulment" is distinct from the common Eastern concept where beings reincarnate by donning and discarding successive earthly vehicles. Aquinas posited "personhood" as dependent on both the "soul" and body. This is an important tenet in Catholicism lest "dualism" disparage physical procreation, the interruption of which was always a "sin" but distinct from "murder." As Jane Hurst, PhD, explains in *The History of Abortion in the Catholic Church*, an immature fetal body was deemed incapable of receiving a "soul." Because the "actualizing principle" can "only be present in a body capable of receiving it," early term abortion did not constitute killing. And it was not until 1869 that Pope Pius IX implied immediate "ensoulment" by proclaiming excommunication for all abortion.

It should be noted that although Papal "infallibility" was also established during the reign of Pius IX, it is of very limited scope and has never encompassed anti-abortion teaching. Some theologians, however, see the current Papacy as attempting to stifle dissent by "upgrading" the contraception/abortion position.

LEGISLATED CATHOLICISM

The debate should hold more than passing interest for United States citizens, so many of whose liberties are influenced by the politicizing of this foreign sovereignty that is the Vatican. For example, the current Catholic position, now absorbed whole cloth by the fundamentalist community, is manifest verbatim in the proposed "human life amendments" endorsed by both Presidents Reagan and Bush. Such measures, though proponents insist they are pro-birth control, would proscribe most effective contraception as "abortifacient" by conveying legal "personhood" on all fertilized eggs (a great number of which are discarded naturally in any event). As has been earlier remarked, this phenomenon is particularly disturbing in that, while the country's citizenry brings a diversity of religious and philosophic perspectives to civil issues, the legislating of particular sectarian tenets flagrantly violates church/ state separation.

PROPAGANDA

With many anti-abortionists it is an article of faith that abortion traumatizes women. But, while depression following childbirth is fairly common, the nation's major medical organizations have explained to the Supreme Court that "women who have abortions are less likely to suffer psychiatric disability than women who are denied abortions." The brief, submitted in defense of choice for the Webster case, also remarks that "the predominant response to abortion is relief" (*New York Times* 4/5/89).

When commissioned to document the fallacy of widespread post-abortion trauma, Reagan's Surgeon General C. Everett Koop actually had to apologize that he was unable to produce findings impugning abortion. "I couldn't find anyone to support what the Reagan Administration thought would be the result of the study," he said (*New York Times* 6/16/89).

THE PARTY LINES

The Attorney General had no such compunction. The 1986 Meese Commission, in service of the Administration's "moral" censorship agenda, shamelessly cited only selected conservatives to conclude, against much mainstream professional opinion, that pornography begets violence. Such insistence is particularly suspect when it is considered that for conservatives the definition of pornography encompasses sex education and AIDS prevention. But Dr. Koop ventured, against the administrative grain, that the best way to reduce abortion incidence would be to upgrade the level of contraception available in this country. And he was utterly reviled for issuing an AIDS report which included words like penis and vagina. "I didn't know what else to call them," the doctor exclaimed (*New York Times* 6/16/89).

New York's pro-reproductive-choice Catholic and Democratic Governor Mario Cuomo was so alarmed by the political emergence of religious agenda that he felt called upon to review "delayed ensoulment" during his church's sustained attack on 1984's pro-choice Vice Presidential candidate Geraldine Ferraro. "Aquinas says it takes six weeks from conception for the soul to make it into a male body and three months into a female body," explained the Governor (*New York Times* 8/14/84). He also declared abortion to be a "matter of the woman's conscience" which should not be subject to such "overwhelmingly male groups" as the Supreme Court and the Congress (New York *Daily News* 9/11/89). But in 1989, the United States Catholic Conference and George Bush filed Court briefs requesting reversal of Roe v. Wade.

AN ASSAULT ON RELIGIOUS FREEDOM

It must indeed be argued that the imposition of one religious belief on all U.S. residents, including members and clergy of other religions, is a dramatic invasion of *their* religious freedom. That many religions are pro-choice is apparent in the membership of the Religious Coalition for Abortion Rights (RCAR), which includes over 30 major national institutions dedicated to religious and reproductive freedom. Their position, as published in 1987, is that "since there is no agreement among the denominations, no one particular dogma should be enacted into law." They believe such attempts constitute a First Amendment assault on religions teaching "that abortion may sometimes be a moral solution to a problem pregnancy." Another RCAR publication, "We Affirm," compiles the strong, unequivocal pro-choice statements of such mainstream religious bastions as the American Ethical Union, the American Jewish Congress, the Episcopal Church, the Presbyterian Church U.S.A., the Union of American Hebrew Congregations, the Unitarian Universalist Association, the United Church of Christ, and the United Methodist Church.

Of course, anti-rights factions arise among pro-choice denominations. But not all evangelicals (Christians focused on spreading the message) are fundamentalist. Some are now formally organized for reproductive rights. There is also great disunity within the ostensibly anti-choice denominations. Catholics For a Free Choice, operating out of Washington, DC, has become a major voice in the escalating dissent among Catholic laity.

THE BIBLE DOES NOT MENTION ABORTION

That fundamentalists, who define themselves by literal readings of the Bible, are anti-abortion exposes a shocking theological deficit. The Bible is totally silent on the subject although abortion, contraception, and infanticide were widely practiced in biblical times to limit family size.

In fact, the earliest Bible-based religion, Judaism, considers the fetus not a person but an attribute of the pregnant woman's body, as is implied in Exodus 21:22-23. This passage describes a miscarriage induced by brawling men as incurring only a fine. The Jewish legal interpretation is that the loss of a fetus does not warrant the "life for life" penalty which would have obtained had a "death" occurred [Zwerin 87]. This distinction between "personhood" and fetal life also derives from Genesis 2:7, which considers a "living being" as one to whom God has imparted breath. Although situations deemed indicative of abortion are widely varied, most U.S. Jewish groups, in firm commitment to separation of church and state, flatly oppose government regulation of abortion.

The fundamentalist characterization of the anti-choice position as scripturally based *Christianity* is even more tortured. In spite of widely reported abortion in contemporaneous Greek and Roman medical literature, the New Testament (the distinctly Christian portion of the Bible) is utterly without reference. Even Paul, a biblical Christian frequently phobic on things sexual, made absolutely no mention of abortion.

In the scriptural vacuum, fundamentalists grasp at inapposite straws, often trotting out Onan, the old seed-spiller, to "document" a position against any contraception. But God "slew" Onan (Genesis 38:8-10) for not impregnating his dead brother's wife, an act demanded by an ingrained tradition called "levirate marriage." Onan immortalized himself, it would seem, more indelibly through coitus interruptus than have others through the reverse. Now the ubiquitous practice of masturbation has become the "sin of onanism" which impugns birth control, abortion, and homosexuality, none of which have anything whatever to do with the matter of not impregnating one's widowed sister-in-law.

The pronatalism implied in such scriptural injunctions to multiply reflects a sparse desert tribe's persistent risk of extinction. Indeed, were the same practicality which informed the biblical policy applied today, it would categorically mandate fertility control.

RANK HYPOCRISY

The anti-abortion movement was eerily foreseen by progressives and conservatives alike. George Orwell's futuristic *1984* (written in 1949) envisioned an Anti-Sex League whose red sash was the "aggressive symbol of chastity." The present zealots' symbol is a red rose but it's the thought that counts. Philosopher/novelist Ayn Rand saw it coming too. A rabid governmental minimalist, she declared herself "profoundly opposed" to Ronald Reagan. "Since he denies the right to abortion, he cannot be a defender of any rights" (*New York Times* obituary 3/7/82).

But with President Reagan and God on their side, the religious right strategized endlessly to suppress in others the sexuality many of their numbers were so spectacularly unable to control in their own lives. As pillars of televangelism like Jimmy Swaggart and

Jimmy Baker repented their sordid little adventures on air, the Alan Guttmacher Institute (7/88) reported that "born-again" Christians accounted for 16% of all abortions. And, perhaps because of the taboo on effective contraception, Catholics showed a higher abortion rate than Protestants.

Then in 1989, against the express advice of a medical advisory panel appointed to study the issue, the Bush Administration extended a Reagan ban on the use of fetal tissue in research for diseases like Parkinson's, Alzheimer's, and diabetes. "It's like the Middle Ages," commented Dr. Birt Harvey, president of the American Academy of Pediatrics (*New York Times* 11/2/89).

Even as the county's prestigious Lasker award was received by Dr. Etienne-Emile Baulieu for developing the abortifacient RU 486, eminent medical experts, including the President's personal physician, were *disqualified* for administration posts because of pro-choice positions and support for in-vitro fertilization research (*New York Times* 10/18/89). And to think this is the President who grandly declared on May 11, 1989: "The days of the dictator are over" (Press Conference on Panama).

The 1989 elections confirmed that a vast pro-choice U.S. majority, complacent under the presumed umbrella of Roe v. Wade, had been rudely awakened by the Webster decision. The '89 Washington march for choice had been half a million strong. "FREE BARBARA BUSH!" they chanted, convinced she'd be down there with them if it weren't for that tiresome husband. Then, major, significant victories for rights candidates moved moderate Congressional Republicans, many of them women, to decry the party's anti-abortion position as an irrational and growing political liability. But the courts were *already* packed, with the Administration held resolutely hostage to the zealots' tax-exempt largess.

A PROTECTION RACKET

No matter what the religionists say, their motive is control. Their premises are not theological postulates, but rather strategies tailored to necessitate protection rackets against "sins" they've defined. The chief victims are, and always have been women, through whose services patriarchies perpetuate themselves. As will be discussed in the following chapter, the monotheistic movement itself was a deliberate campaign against extant gender-balanced and matrifocal religions. And crusades were waged against "heretics" who dared imply a female aspect to divinity.

The global roots of the issue surfaced briefly in the Iranian Ayatollah's reaction to Salman Rushdie's "blaspheming" the Muslim religion by reviving a "discredited" scripture. *The Satanic Verses* refers to a passage wherein Mohammed recognized three *goddesses* (*New York Times* 2/23/89). Here, a passing glance at the idea of female divinity warranted a Khomeini death contract.

The subtlety of Western patriarchs effects death just as sure. In a total exclusion of women, the Catholic hierarchy makes illegal abortion the leading cause of pregnancy-related death in Latin America. There theocracy entirely precludes safe reproductive control. Hoping to expand this virulence, the United States' bishops proclaimed in 1989: "No Catholic can responsibly take a 'pro-choice' stand when the 'choice' in question involves the taking of innocent human life." The bishops also "consider" excommunication for rights activists. Meanwhile, Catholics and fundamentalists alike delete, from such AIDS education as is permitted, all allusion specific to young gay males, many of whom will die from HIV infection, but whose very mention constitutes "pornography."

By day the religionists hammer and shove women trying to get in to their gynecologists; by night they burn clinics to the ground. As Randall Terry, inspired leader of the "Operation Rescue" clinic blockades remarked: "I don't think Christians should use birth control. You consummate your marriage as often as you like — and if you have babies, you have babies."

ONE FAMILY'S NIGHTMARE

Compared to some "conservative" activism, clinic bombings are rather diffuse. One "right-to-life" group zeroed in on a comatose Long Island woman whose family sought to improve her chances of survival through pregnancy termination. A claim of "fetal guardianship" necessitated multiple court appearances and significantly delayed the hospital's performance of an abortion which eventually helped revive the woman in question (*New York Times* 1/12/90).

Here the "pro-life" enthusiasts wrought a judicial nightmare for a family on the brink of physical and emotional disaster. They simply would not take "no" for an answer and appealed every decision that came down. It is now not uncommon for women to have to squeeze in abortions between favorable court decisions and the appeal of those decisions on behalf of "fetuses' rights." Such is the extent of theocratic incursion in the United States today.

BIOLOGISM

Fundamentalists want easy answers and easy validity. They are of superior species (*not evolved* from apelike primates), and they immeasurably surpass the sinners against whose ground they feature themselves in holy relief. In another time they executed proponents of heliocentricity, its seeming blasphemous that their earth not be the center of the universe. And in a kind of dogmatism of the biologic, they confuse the protoplasm that is substance with the consciousness that is the essence of personhood.

In secular terms this "biologism" contends that a fertilized egg contains all genetic information peculiar to an adult body. Of course, so does a hangnail. This does not avail either of the self-awareness characterizing personhood.

Because acorns are not oak trees, most scientists come down firmly on the "not a person" side. Genetic biology shows that physical structure (hands, nose, etc.) and reflexive capability widely precede the cerebral development upon which consciousness is predicated. And genetic researcher Charles A. Gardner writes that early embryos are not even completely ordained as distinct *physical* phenomena. Sometimes "two sibling embryos combine into one," he explains. "If the two original embryos were determined to become particular individuals, such a thing could not happen." Recognizing themselves to be "different people" they "would not unite." Gardner continues: "Time itself must be woven into the fabric of the embryo before it becomes a baby (*The Nation* 11/13/89).

THE SILENT SCAM

Such information has no effect whatever upon the shameless "right-to-life" propagandists. In 1985, several prominent fetal experts assembled to exposé "The Silent Scream," a video of a 12-week abortion featuring a fetus purportedly recoiling in pain. The footage, which was actually being touted by the White House, turned out to be in slow motion until the abortion at which point the tape was accelerated to imply purposeful action. The physicians, all recommended by the American College of Obstetricians and Gynecologists, explained that because the cerebral cortex, which perceives pain, does not yet function at the stage of development in question, any fetal activity was purely reflexive (*New York Times* editorial 3/11/85).

But deaf to science, theology, and reason, the theocrats persevere, as if choosing to give birth should be undertaken more lightly than choosing not to. They eschew the oddity of 200,000 world-wide annual botched abortion deaths; some of which dying are rejected by medical facilities fearing they may run afoul of the U.S.A.'s Mexico City Policy (*New York Times* 2/27/89). And they reserve for themselves the right to plan the families of everyone in the world.

THE DECISION TO REMAIN FERTILE

In the United States any adult who wishes can be legally sterilized (with a few states requiring spousal consent). In fact, the health risks and expenses attending contraception available here have made sterilization the country's most common birth control choice, practiced widely even among women still in their 20s [Guttmacher 3/88]. In this context it can be argued that any woman facing a problem pregnancy has implied a rather noble and generous *decision to remain fertile*. For this social option, one would expect pronatalists to thank the women in question. But the country's religionists discourage the decision to remain fertile with their insistence on enforcing the time and situation of reproduction. And if the elimination of abortion as a backup option makes United States birth control even more unreliable, many more women, some of whom will later regret their decisions, will undergo sterilization.

Roe v. Wade itself is presumptuously invasive in its permission for third term state regulation on behalf of a fetus, as if a theoretical potential for survival entitles any being to commandeer a person's vital systems. Even *presuming* "personhood," persons are not *required* to sustain life for other persons. One *might* rescue another from a fire, but is certainly not legally compelled to do so. And by no code may an individual commandeer the biosystems of another, unless, of course, the anti-rights minority is now willing to impose mandated parental organ donating to the born as well as the "unborn."

Nature, in choosing women for the responsibility of procreation, apparently also included a motive to control this fertility. Imprisonment through the reproductive capacity is a profound denigration of women's faculty. The near exclusive "moral" agency of men has thus far produced several millennia of global conflict, an environment exhausting the resources necessary to sustain its people, a population time bomb approaching six billion, and a nuclear capability which could make all these issues irreversibly moot. That women, in such a context, be presumed as moral agents is a moral "good" if not a moral mandate. That fertilized eggs be endowed with legal standing is an insult to the moral agency of all women.

Women do not abort viable or late pregnancies whimsically, if for no other reason than to do so is infinitely more complicated and expensive than to abort early. But contingencies do arise. Some anomalies cannot be detected until the 16-20 week period. Restricting abortion of such fetuses effectively removes childbearing as an option for "at risk" parents who would not attempt conception if forced to carry an anomaly to term. And whatever the contingency, be it an imminent nuclear war or an AIDS fetus, it is not for the government to impose childbirth on the women involved.

Historians, law professors, and the American Medical Association, along with a host of other major medical and professional groups, filed briefs in defense of Roe when the Reagan/Bush Justice Department requested its overturn in Webster. And although self-determination should in no way be predicated upon the will of the majority, as it happens, the majority here *is* pro-choice. Consistent polls show margins of at least 2 to 1 holding abortion as the exclusive province of the women in question, e.g., the Media General/Associated Press Poll (New York *Daily News* 7/24/89) and the *New York Times*/CBS News Poll *(New York Times* 8/3/89). The anti-rights packed courts in no way represent majority constituent views of the elected officials who appoint judges. Rather they reflect the political accommodation of a financially substantial minority. It is tragic that this judicial legacy will pervade the first quarter of the next century. And President Bush's appointment, Justice David H. Souter, to replace Supreme Court rights bulwark Justice William Brennan (retired in 1990) will, quite simply, define lives of over half the people in the United States.

WE ARE THE PEOPLE!

Choice does not impose its morality on those who disagree. They are free to carry to term and to preach about the goodness of doing so. Conversely, anti-rights advocates wish to impose their views on all others, including those whose religious and moral convictions preclude random and irresponsible reproduction. Many women feel it is immoral to bring into the world a child they can neither love nor clothe. "Choose life!" the clinic terrorists scream. But how can one choose anything if the faculty for choice is itself foreclosed?

Rights advocates are "extremist" only to those who do not understand the extremism of the opposition. It is extremely important not to have one's capacity to love co-opted by the government in service of compulsory reproduction. And each passing year renders the 18-year commitment of motherhood more expensive, with items and services that did not even exist in the recent past surfacing regularly as "necessities."

When "stridency" for choice is censured, it should be noted that state seizure of its female citizens for nine month hitches in involuntary incubative servitude warrants some stridency. If men were suddenly struck pregnant, test tube gestation and government child rearing would be universal within a decade. And without the stridency of decades past, the women of neither side would have the right to vote.

CHAPTER 6

RELIGION

"God made Adam and Eve, not Adam and Steve," exclaimed the Suffolk rights opponents, implying that the most ancient recorded histories would shore up their prejudice. Televised sandwich boards reaffirm the homophobic sentiment from the protest sidelines of most gay pride parades. "Did She?" enquired an interested onlooker.

WHOSE GOD WROTE GENESIS?

While there exists a vast diversity in interpretation of the mythologies fundamentalists cite to justify their anti-gay/anti-woman legislative agenda, by absolutely no stretch of the imagination does the Genesis account of Adam and Eve originate with the biblical god or with the monotheistic presumption thereof. That a literal representation of this legend be presumed as basis for Constitutional law, which indeed it now is by many powerful religionists, would be far beyond the ridiculous as fiction. Things being as they are, however, contemporary United States libertarians must toil through Eden's garden in search of civil rights.

And, in a more general vein, all Westerners must there trudge because Genesis, the first book of the Bible, has become a subliminal permeation, almost universally invoked to explain and maintain the extant hierarchal male/female structure. In short, Adam and Eve authorize men's control of women, and document that domination to a male god as divine revelation. This taint ranges from the impugnation of "Adam and Steve" to the extraordinary idea of childbirth's pain as woman's punishment for *her* sexual sin. It should be remembered that it is Eve, and not Adam, who inspires "sin" having had truck with "the serpent." And by biblical times, the serpent itself had experienced radical transformation from its Pagan association with "wisdom" to a biblical connotation of "evil."

First came Adam. Then, as an afterthought, Eve was derived from his rib. In mechanical obeisance to this garden "order of things," presented in the earliest of formative years as the way the world came about, little boys reject toys and blue jeans used by girls as contaminated with "cooties," and Catholic men deny women any participation whatever in their global hierarchy. Let there be no question at all that Adam and Eve are important tools in the business of sexism. The *New Catholic Encyclopedia* (under "Genesis, Book of") cheerfully describes Genesis as "the source for many basic doctrines of the Judeo-Christian religion" including "doctrines of original sin."

ADAM AND EVE WERE PAGAN

This kind of credibility is, of course, what fundamentalists sense they lose to Darwinian evolution. And in light of the extraordinary patriarchal propagandizement of the issue, the mythology of Genesis must be exhumed and some central points made: Adam and Eve are Pagan in origin; in much early mythology females created males, as would be the obvious conclusion of the primitive peoples who originated these scenarios; and many biblical accounts reflect the overthrow of gender balanced and matrifocal systems whose demise began with the discovery of paternity and was accelerated in Judeo-Christianity:

Adapa was the Sumerian "adam," the term "adapa" being a generic referent to the mythological model for a new race being developed by the Mother Goddess NIN.TI (Lady of Life). The purpose of the "adapa" was to till the soil for an assembly of gods, male and female. The biblical parallel is underlined by the fact that in Sumerian "TI" means both "life" and "rib," a phenomenon highly evocative of the more recent Eve's emergence from Adam's rib. Another parallel is that the number seven was of persistent mystical significance to the Pagans. One early Mesopotamian account actually relates creation in seven tablets, a feature Genesis's "seven days" may reflect.

A unique treatment of this matter proceeds from Zecharia Sitchin, who presents the radical theory that these mythologies reflect the workings of ancient off-world (extraterrestrial) scientists experimenting with the developing earthly primates. Although Sitchin's direction is highly unconventional, his detailed and meticulous exploration in *The 12th Planet* is rooted in translations by the past century's most orthodox Near East scholars. The mythologies themselves are there, no doubt about it. And it is fact, not theory that those Pagan texts dramatically predate the Genesis accounts, authorship of which is placed in the first millennium BCE (Before the Common Era).

CLASSIC DOCUMENTATION

Under "Cosmogony" the *Interpreter's Dictionary of the Bible* flatly describes the "Old Testament" creation stories as "based upon traditional ancient Near Eastern lore." The *New Catholic Encyclopedia* reports that it is "commonly accepted by Catholic scholars" and "in general accord with official Catholic teaching" that the narrative vehicle of the first eleven chapters of Genesis is from "extra-Biblical sources that antedate Israel," the "likeliest" geographic origin of which is "Northern Mesopotamia."

Distinguished mythologist Joseph Campbell enthusiastically concurs as to this material's pre-biblical antiquity. He cites archeological evidence, to place the earliest maiden/serpent myths "somewhere in the neighborhood of 7,500 BC" with these in turn based on older matriarchal lore concurrent "with the first appearance of Homo sapiens on the prehistoric scene." And throughout what is now Europe, copious statuary evidence of Mother Goddess worship, traditionally dismissed as "cult-related," can be dated as early as 25,000 BCE with sites of such ceremonies as old as 30,000 BCE [Stephenson 81].

Creation stories are told and retold in prebiblical Mesopotamian cosmology, where matriarchal or mixed-gendered deities mold, often from clay, beings who eventually wind up in a flood. The biblical "Noah" story has multiple Pagan forerunners, the best known of which is a Babylonian "Epic of Gilgamesh."

While most traditional scholars place the origins of these legends in Sumerian tradition [Von Rad 61], one persevering soul, Colonel James Churchward, spent his entire life linguistically tracing the ubiquitous flood mythologies to a common cosmology in a proposed sunken Pacific continent. And a more contemporary linguist, grandson to the famous founder of the Berlitz school of languages, puts the common culture in Plato's sunken Atlantis. Charles Berlitz has gone so far as to catalogue archeological evidence of the ancient underwater Atlantic ruins which lend credence to his theories.

Now NIN.TI is forgotten, and with her a host of heavenly sisters. As was earlier discussed, what happened to these matriarchs was that the discovery of a male role in conception triggered a regulation of women through enforced fidelity. Thus men came to own children and women much as they did agrarian goods. Or as Will Durant explained of these times: "the male now demanded [from women] that fidelity which he thought would enable him to pass on his accumulations to children presumably his own."

SEXISM DIGNIFIED BY RELIGION

Religion, of course, reflected and eventually "explained" this development in an upheaval of divine personages, plainly relating the destruction of the female as prerequisite to the ascension of the males. In Babylonia's seven tablets it is well described how Marduk gained his godly kingship through the slaying of Ti[amat], the Mother Goddess. Or as Durant put it: "The gods, who had been mostly feminine, became great bearded patriarchs . . ."

The Pagan roots do emerge in analysis of Judeo/Christian texts. For example, "Elohim," a common scriptural term for God, is a Hebrew pluralization of the goddess Eloh's name. And the mechanics of the Matriarch's demise are indeed blatantly documented in that selective collection of multi-source, multi-lingual translations which eventually came to be compiled as the Bible. Most female deities were erased in being as well as gender, subsumed, even in their destruction, as just so many "false gods." It was in the interest of "monotheizing" that these purges proceeded. And the god in whose service monotheization persevered was a jealous, childlike, murderous male into whose mouth rules were put for imprisoning women through their reproductive capacities.

DESTROY THEIR NAMES!

The Bible is awash with injunctions to demolish every trace of Pagan cites, cultures, and persons. Throughout, God and his agents slay, burn, and wreak havoc upon the slightest and most incomprehensible of provocations. Take, for example, Deuteronomy 12:2-3, wherein is mandated the destruction of "all the places where the nations whom you shall dispossess served their gods," with instructions to tear down altars, dash pillars, burn Asherim, "hew down the graven images of their gods, and destroy their name out of that place." Small wonder a degree of historic invisibility has befallen the Mother God.

And such grand female divines as bit the patriarchal dust in this transition! Consider, for instance, Lilith, once called the "hand" of Inanna, Heaven's Queen. Lilith emerged in Hebrew literature as Adam's first wife who, deeming herself man's equal, declined to lie beneath Adam. Feminist researcher Merlin Stone has explored such revisions in some detail. But what eventually occurred is that Lilith was reduced to a "demon" who stole men's seed to conjur "illegimate" children.

As a final blow, the Pagan stories were rewritten to reflect cosmic creation by a male god and this as though it were "revealed" word as old as time. This edition, of course, is what now presents itself as Genesis, subject of nationwide litigation for mandated inclusion as science in the public schools.

COMMENTS

"It's the word of God!" the faithful scream. And they vote. And they send in money. And they are a major presence in U.S. politics today. No matter what *should* be happening vis-à-vis church/state separation, these religionists' influence is being felt in every arena of our country's government from the Suffolk Legislative Auditorium to the United States Supreme Court.

As a grassroots activist, my experience is that many of the rank and file theocrats are profoundly ignorant, and that the reason for this is that thinking and educated citizens are afraid to talk to them. U.S. consensus tends to grant "diplomatic immunity" to religious zealots in the delusion that religious freedom means freedom from honest dialogue as well as from governmental intrusion. I have asked fundamentalists in what language the Bible was written and some have replied: "English." In the face of their explicit anti-Semitism I have submitted that Jesus was Jewish. In response I was accused of "blasphemy." I have ventured that Adam and Eve were not real people and the woman with whom I was speaking made a sign behind her back so that a friend would interrupt us. I have also received, with some regularity, menacing communications as documented to Leviticus. One was signed "anonymous" but contained a return address.

I think we must begin a theological dialogue. It is one thing to respect another's religious beliefs. But when one's neighbors publicly certify their faiths to refutable errors and lies, I believe it is irresponsible to "pass" on the issues. I believe individual freedoms in the United States of America would not be so imperiled as they are today had a dialogue transpired on religious matters in the openness afforded other subjects. But in fact, the mainstream has hardly spoken to the fundamentalists since the Scopes trial. And now they are dictating national party platforms in the name of moral consensus.

Neither history nor theology regards the text of Genesis as the literal revealed word of the monotheists' male god. Literalistic biblical interpretations are particular sectarian perspectives, and as such not suitable for legislation in the United States. Let us repeat this early and often, on the talk shows and in letters to the editor across this country until it is, to hope for the very least, noted. And let us remember that a perfectly respectable reply to a report that "God made Adam and Eve, not Adam and Steve" is "No, She made everyone."

MISTRANSLATIONS

Through specific scriptural interpretations, the same standards that promote stability in heterosexual relationships have become agents of its destruction among gays. But now a significant number of biblical scholars has explored the errata called upon to justify this consummate violence upon the men and women of the gay community.

For some Pagans considered sex an act of worship. And passages implying "prostitution" may sometimes reflect a priestly characterization of male and female participation in such sexual rites. Whatever the practices' context, however, several scriptural terms now translated to connote homosexuality per se originally denoted prostitutes — homosexual and heterosexual. Mistranslations also befell words meaning "soft," "loose," and "sacred." But as is remarked by John Boswell (Professor of History at Yale University and winner of the 1981 American Book Awards for History) in his exhaustive treatment of these matters: "In spite of misleading English translations which may imply the contrary, the word 'homosexual' does not occur in the Bible: no extant text or manuscript, Hebrew, Greek, Syriac, or Aramaic, contains such a word."

NO GAYS AT SODOM

Perhaps the most spectacular revelation is that the incident at Sodom, a town which has now sacrificed its name to the impugnation of gay people, has been shown through modern scholarship to involve not homosexuality but rather inhospitality and possibly gang rape. The divine travelers (angels of the Lord, as it were) may have fallen victim to the Near East practice of "humiliating and demasculinizing a conquered enemy by treating him 'like a woman.'" In fact, Auburn Theological Seminary's Professor of Biblical Interpretation, Dr. Walter Wink, said just that in an exposition on "Biblical Perspectives on Homosexuality."

This "Sodom" passage, in Genesis 19, describes a scene where a mob outside Lot's door demands to "know" his guests. Lot placidly offers them his virgin daughters, but unpacified, the mob insists upon Lot's guests. The context here is patently of violence, rather than love.

But there is even serious controversy about whether the Hebrew word translated "to know" was actually intended in sexual context. The term appears scripturally many times in a purely cerebral syntax. Several scholars now point out that in biblical times the passage was not interpreted to concern sexual sin, and that the mob may have meant merely to learn who these strangers under Lot's roof might be. What is very clear, however, beyond any shadow of a doubt, is that the passage has nothing whatever to do with consensual relationships.

LEVITICUS

As for biblical passages that do definitely have to do with gay sex, the book of Leviticus is the only Hebrew scriptural (called by Christians "Old Testament") source. But this material is certainly not germane for Christians, nor indeed, for most contemporary Jews. Judaism itself was never monolithic. And that certain strains of a flexible oral tradition came to be set down in print did not render them universally or unendingly binding. The primary intent of much Levitical law was to effect religious distinction. The priests of those times were intent to distinguish themselves from the Near East Pagan neighbors. And to this end did they design elaborate dietary and ritualistic restrictions as indicative of cultural purity but *not of moral law*. Leviticus enumerates these minutiae, and among them, preceded in the same chapter by explicit injunctions that the people of Israel not walk in the statutes of the Pagan Egyptians and Canaanites, is the oft cited Leviticus 18:22: "You shall not lie with a male as with a woman; it is an abomination." The ubiquitous death penalty is attached in Leviticus 20:13.

SELECTIVE THEOCRACY

One can certainly not selectively assume contemporary moral (let alone legislative) relevance for two sentences of this book while ignoring the rest of Leviticus. And the book, in total, addresses itself predominantly to the specific parts of flayed bulls and where in the temple to place these in relation to an altar. The ritual uncleanliness, which was designated by the term now translated "abomination," is applied serendipitously to menstruating women, rock badgers, and males who ate of the blessed bulls on the third day after the flaying. Also impugned are the lame, the blind, the blemished, the facially mutilated (described in some translations as persons with flat noses), dwarfs, and the damaged of testicle, any of which individuals would "profane" the sanctuaries. Would the fundamentalists like to implement these provisions as well?

Midway through the book, God kills Aaron's sons for offering a religiously incorrect fire. Death is then mandated for a great many erotic experiences including sex with beasts (all parties here should perish) and ménages à trois among husbands, wives and mothers-in-law. Toward the end of the book, explicit permission is granted for the taking of slaves from among Pagans and sojourning strangers, with specific designation of same as bequeathable property.

Now many contemporary Jewish leaders emphatically reject literalistic interpretations of the scriptures their ancient ancestors authored. As Rabbi Yoel H. Kahn of San Francisco said of the "anti-gay" passage: "Why only on this verse do we become fundamentalists? We haven't been afraid to dissent from Leviticus before" (*New York Times* 6/26/90). The occasion was the Central Conference of American Rabbis' decision to endorse acknowledged, sexually active lesbians and gay men to the Reform Jewish rabbinate.

That present day Christians would be invoking Leviticus against gays (and they have done, from Anita Bryant right on up) is truly bizarre. The New Testament, the definitively Christian portion of the Bible, emphasizes a mission of experiential or mystical awakening to a "kingdom of heaven" within, not sought through particular physical restrictions. Christianity's founder was a Jewish mystic who taught enlightenment through esoteric (inner) rather than exoteric (doctrinal) practice. And he went out of his way to defy the external restrictions, eschewing the traditional fasts, flagrantly harvesting or healing on the sabbath, setting "a man against his father, and a daughter against her mother" (Matthew 10:35), and teaching "as one who had authority" (Matthew 7:29) rather than respectfully citing scriptural precedent, as did the traditional rabbis.

Nor was Jesus simply indifferent about these restrictions. He was at times flagrantly hostile: "I have not come to bring peace, but a sword" (Matthew 10:34). *That's why he was always in so much trouble.* And he went so far as to describe the lawgivers as actual impediments to enlightenment: "woe to you, scribes and Pharisees, hypocrites! because you shut the kingdom of heaven against men;

for you neither enter yourselves, nor allow those who would enter to go in" (Matthew 23:13).

PAUL—A CONVERT

As for clear New Testament references which might concern Christians, there is but Paul's letter to the Romans. And the Romans passage, like the material in Leviticus, must be considered as to source. For in 20th century U.S.A., Paul would be well on his way to an institution. He was, it would seem, before his eccentric Christian "conversion," something of a holy terror, blandly overseeing persecutions, including stonings to death, of Christians.

Notwithstanding this sectarian shift of gears, Paul had been steeped in a lifetime of exoteric indoctrination and entertained much ambivalence about sex. But even Paul, in his unemphasized and brief remark on things gay, was both confusing and confused. He considers same-gender relations symbolically, as a consequence visited upon heterosexuals because of their theological transgressions. Romans 1 explains that: "because they exchanged the truth about God for a lie and worshipped and served the creature rather than the Creator . . . For this reason God gave them up to dishonorable passions. Their women exchanged natural relations for unnatural, and the men likewise gave up natural relations with women and were consumed with passion for one another, men committing shameless acts with men and receiving in their own persons the due penalty for their error." Perhaps unaware of homosexuality as an orientation, Paul regards the apparently rather excessive appetites of the individuals in question as externally superimposed, over those persons' innate heterosexualities, by a God jealous of being less served than mammon.

Nor would the assessment (of same-sex appetites construed as their own recrimination) be altogether surprising in a context where male rape of other males was wielded as a degradation for despised and conquered enemies.

But, of course, the distorted perspective, in and of itself, absolutely precludes reference to mutual loving. Concurrently Paul erroneously awaited an imminent coming of a physical "kingdom," from which any relationships might distract the faithful: "he who marries . . . does well; and he who refrains from marriage will do better'' (1 Corinthians 7:38). His predominant attitude here is that marriage is a safeguard against "temptation." But elsewhere, in the same chapter, he specifies that advice he is giving on sex is his own and not of "the Lord."

So Paul's remark altogether ignores same-gender orientation. And the only other New Testament "references" number among those terms which are now translated to impugn homosexuality, but which contemporary scholars like Wink and Boswell explain referred most probably to prostitution and other phenomena distinct from "homosexuality." This leaves Christian scripture basically silent on the subject.

PARABLES

In general, Jesus spoke to the "multitudes" in "parables" related to daily life. He did not expect to be understood by everyone but by "only those to whom it is given" (Matthew 19:11) to understand. And the little word-pictures had the advantage of memorability and subtle transmission. Also, their obscurity to the faithless would provide a certain degree of insulation against inevitable transcriptional tampering. Of course, another advantage to obliqueness was that, on the surface, a parable could appear to agree with the adversaries' legal code and permit three years of ministry before arrest and execution. The sexual images were almost always symbolic, as with Matthew 25's five foolish "maidens" who showed up at the wedding with no lamp oil and consequently lost out to another five that brought their own supply. The "kingdom of heaven" exacts one's own illumination, and not that of another.

Other parables warn against adulterating the new mysticism with the old external structure through a metaphor of pouring new wine into old wineskins (Matthew 9:17). As new wine would expand to destroy the skins and spill the wine, so would the new teaching be inappropriately stored in the extant moral rubric. It is even sometimes argued that all the sexual references are metaphors for spiritual matters, with "divorce" and "infidelity" representing estrangement from one's own spiritual integrity.

But the anti-gay sentiment does not come from Jesus of Nazareth. And although Paul subscribed to it, he did so from habit, from indoctrination, from a belief in an imminent millennium, or from elsewhere. Paul, in all likelihood, never met the earthly Jesus. And the Gospel authors, Matthew, Mark, Luke, and John (several of whom most probably knew their teacher well), make no mention of things or persons lesbian and gay. Predictably, the fundamentalists' legislative agenda pays full service to Paul's homophobia but ignores his injunction in 1 Corinthians 14:34 that women should remain silent in church.

THE GNOSTIC GOSPELS

Recent discoveries have shed some long overdue light on the New Testament in general. The Gnostic Gospels (gnostic meaning "directly knowing") were unearthed in upper Egypt in 1945. What is truly amazing is that the fundamentalist Christians, by self-definition obsessed with scripture, have scarcely noticed these newly emerged accounts of their leader's life and teachings, some of which serious scholars date as contemporaneous with or earlier than the New Testament Gospels.

Published in readable English compilation [Robinson 77], many of these texts, probably hidden by monks avoiding the hierarchal church's purges of "heresy," were "heretical" precisely because they ignored the church and taught awakening through inner mystical work independent of priestly councils and their prescriptions. Much of the material also presumes an androgynous godhead and includes members of both genders as full teaching participants. Skeptics querying the resistance any given priesthood might have offered such texts should recall that a "testament" itself (old or new), considered as to Latin derivation, is a covenant sworn upon one's balls.

THE OTHER MARY

In another potentially "heretical" gnostic feature, Mary Magdalene emerges as a disciple rather than a groupie. And in the Gnostic Gospel of Mary Magdalene, Jesus explicitly instructs the disciples:

"Do not lay down any rules beyond what I appointed for you, and do not give a law like the lawgiver lest you be constrained by it."

Still another gnostic earmark was an emphasis on the transcendence of "ignorance," rather than "sin," as essential to spiritual development. As eminent religious historian Professor Elaine Pagels explains: "Both gnosticism and psychotherapy value, above all, knowledge — the self-knowledge which is insight." Absent such awareness, Pagels continues, there is sustained a "sense of being driven by impulses" one does not understand. Perhaps such a perspective of directly known self-awareness will provide a transition to the New Age.

CHAPTER 7

METAPHYSICS

Contemporary Western culture expects objective resolutions for conflicts which are essentially metaphysical in nature. But doctrine *creates* rather than *resolves* that literalism of the biologic which underlies these disputes. Most of the world's people and all of its mystics have presumed spiritual dimensions beyond the biologic. Whether such phenomena are considered in the Western context of "afterlife" or in the eastern tradition of progressing physical "incarnations," a transcendent "soul" or "entity" is posited.

A divergence in opinion characterized early Christian discussion regarding "resurrection" after death and whether this would involve the physical body or a spiritual representation of same. Many gnostics came down on the latter side, but they lost to the "biologics." Some Christian denominations still await a literal fleshy emergence from the grave for deceased believers. Other faiths walk a blurry line, acknowledging "soul" but as somehow begun in physical being.

OVERSOULS

New Age "revelations," none of which are any more or less documentable than biblical prophesies, are said to be "transmitted" by overarching "entities" who transcend their earthly existences to "remember" individual incarnations, relationships, and genders, in the larger perspective of connectedness to Source. Some of the propositions thus "revealed" form an interesting east/west philosophic bridge, certain trusses of which are directly relevant to contemporary holy war issues. Such perspectives carry with them great energies, and offer refreshing alternatives to the endless duality posed by the literal religions. For example, the "channeled" communicant Emmanuel contends that "no soul is ever destroyed" and that "when a soul chooses to be born, it will be born." He continues: "The soul is wise and would not inhabit a body if it were not to come to term" [Rodegast 85].

Literalists' deepest premises are often of just such a "soul," which precedes earthly life and might indeed suffer eternal discomfort should it misread its labyrinthine scriptural instructions. Even the bravest of Bible belters will concede that a corpse is distinct from a person, being absent that constituent of "soul" which distinguishes the living. What *is there* in live persons and *is not there* among the dead, is the "personhood" whose physicalization demands some major degree of higher brain activity.

Indeed, the literalists' reductionistic notion of "personhood" as protoplasmic activity absent conscious capacity would, if applied across the board, engage half the country's medical resources in circulating blood and breath for the "brain dead." As it is, many resources are already engaged in maintaining those in persistent vegetative states, often against the express wishes of those most closely involved. Nor is potential inhabitation of a biological structure the same as actual occupancy. We do not, for example, mandate freezing of the dead in event their forms may someday be reoccupied through advanced technology.

BIOLOGICAL TYRANNY

Of course, women are not respirators and feeding tubes such as might sustain the uninhabited forms of the "brain dead." Rather they are living, thinking, sentient beings with works, aspirations, and perhaps cancer cures on their agendas. Respirators do not have such goals. Women do. And for women, every conceivable area of life, dignity, spirit, solvency, and future is predicated upon the *ability to choose* whether or not they indeed wish to perform as respirators, heart pumps, and eventually guardians of 18 years' tenure.

In this context, dogmatism of the biologic constitutes a tyranny such as has occasioned the great revolutions of history. In this spiritual perspective it is as intrinsically "American" to argue that childbearing remain voluntary as it is to decry taxation without representation.

A SPIRITUAL PERSPECTIVE

In some metaphysical outlooks, an aborting woman is directing an incoming soul to a more welcomed environment or more opportune season. She is not destroying a soul but rerouting it to the advantage of all parties concerned. But many anti-choicers seem to imagine that those immortal souls about whom they profess such fervent obsession are, in the sole circumstance of abortion, struck suddenly mortal to perish with fertilized eggs they might have occupied. Do these religionists really believe that the billions of fertilized eggs which are discarded naturally represent a universe of eternally lost beings? Should not these questions be asked?

What of the women who know or have reason to suspect that the fetuses they are carrying are seriously malformed or diseased? Continued, of course, such pregnancies produce individuals deserving utmost respect for lives some mystics explain as boldly chosen learning challenges. But many prospective mothers feel it is categorically wrong to facilitate such painful existences. Surely the being entrusted with a disadvantaged person's care, often for the rest of her life, should have final say about extending the invitation. Surely the woman experiencing the pregnancy knows best whether or not it is appropriate. Surely *her* faculties, rather than the President's, should be engaged to decide if an "anencephalitic" fetus (without a brain) is to be carried to term or not.

The fetus is, because of its unique position, quite simply *no body's business* in excess of the pregnant woman's permission. If legislators and the packed courts feel that it is, perhaps research should be directed toward implanting fertilized eggs in the abdominal cavities of men so that they too may enjoy the phenomenon of mandated gestation.

DEATH IMPELS A PRO-CHOICE ESTABLISHMENT

Movement is indeed possible. In recent U.S. history, maternity wards awash with mutilated and dying women induced strong pro-choice sentiment in a medical community which had earlier initiated criminalization. What will it take to move the larger patriarchy? An airborne HIV? A continent dead of starvation? If the patriarchs of the world do not now permit fertility control they will surely mandate it soon. This planet simply cannot sustain its present rate of increase. And of course, the U.S.A.'s new-found pronatal evangelism has quite some antecedent in compulsory sterilization of the "mentally disabled," a category amid which representatives of racial minorities were "diagnosed" in staggering numbers.

GENDER POLITICS

Vis-à-vis gays, biologic dogmatism constitutes a socio/legal enforcement against being oneself. Beings on this planet are literally defined by gendered proclivities and by whom they love. To impose, in the name of biological gender, an unwanted script on the psyche of any person is a kind of assault, this of spirit rather than of vehicle. Societal homophobia pits the instinct of survival, economic and social, diametrically against the instinct to love. And a harsher, more insoluble conflict could not be devised.

New Age perspectives have arisen also upon matters gay. Jane Roberts' revelations through the "voice" of "Seth" devote much discussion to same-sex orientation, and specifically include lesbian and gay male relationships as natural and "valid" expressions of the "biologically necessary" life force of "love" without which "there is no physical commitment to life—no psychic hold." The passage includes a sound condemnation of gender role and heterosexuality constructs, with a particular horror of the violence inherent in males' learned separation of love and sexuality: "This great division has led to your major wars" [Roberts 79]. The discourse also presumes a "natural bisexuality," recognition of which would help resolve "violence and acts or murder."

BEING TRANSCENDS GENDER

Jane Roberts (as Seth) remarks: "A great artist in any field or in any time instinctively feels a private personhood that is greater than the particular sexual identity. As long as you equate identity with your sexuality, you will limit the potentials of the individual and of the species." In a further discussion of homosexuality and religion it is remarked: "There are 'lost' portions of the Bible having to do with sexuality, and with Christ's beliefs concerning it, that were considered blasphemous and did not come down to you through history.'' Such intimations call to mind the suppressed gnostic "heresies.'' And even conventional sources like Paul give credence to these transcendent strains: "There is neither Jew nor Greek, there is neither slave nor free, there is neither male nor female,'' he declares in Galatians 3, "for you are all one in Christ Jesus.''

CROSS-GENDERED HEALERS

The element of gender transcendence in spiritual awakening is an enduring theme in *esoteric* tradition. Throughout history mysticism, healing, and divination have been often presumed among the cross-gendered. The ancient Tarot deck has long tradition as esoterica coded for disguise and preservation in the times of orthodox purges. It shows the end of a "Fool's" journey in the perfection of a "World" card, depicting a dancing breasted figure, veiled below the waist. It is often read that the end of all knowledge is a hermaphrodite with the floating veil hiding the truth.

Transgenderism permeated many early religious cultures. As was mentioned, the Pagans' heterosexual and homosexual religious rights occasioned such chagrin among the monotheistic priests as survives even in contemporary scripture. And in some Near Eastern cultures, males involved with religion would cross-dress, sometimes even castrating themselves to approximate matriarchal divinity [Greenberg 86]. Do not echoes of this tradition survive in today's celibate, cross-dressed Catholic priesthood? And in North America "berdaches," as the French traders termed cross-dressing homosexuals among the native tribes, were respected and often greatly honored as priests and healers.

Today, many mainstream religious denominations position themselves firmly on the side of equal civil rights for gays. Several also expressly authorize the admission of openly lesbian/gay clergy, among them the United Church of Christ, the Unitarian Universalists, and Reform Judaism. In other groups around the country debates proceed on ordination of open gays and blessings for same-gender unions. Meanwhile, such events do transpire locally in disregard of denomination policies.

Someday the extraordinary numbers of closeted gays among the clergy of all denominations may effect awakenings about the historical and mystical centrality of the trans-gendered. Until such time as that, much gay religious work will proceed largely unacknowledged or under such auspices as the explicitly gay Metropolitan Community Churches and the various lesbian and gay synagogues. There are, however, contemporary mystics who feel the *only* mission of gays is to mediate and bridge male and female energies for the healing of this planet; and that lesbians and gay men will always feel hollow absent their conscious recognition of this function [Wright 82].

AIDS AND METAPHYSICS

In December of 1989 the author "interviewed" Whitefeather, an "entity" representing a sisterhood of Native American and Eastern shamans. I was interested in discussing, face to face with a New Age source, the premise, honored in much esoteric tradition, that through distinctions in our consciousness we manifest various symptoms and traumas for our own edification. A current reiteration of this presumption has sustained some criticism from those who interpret its relevance to AIDS as a guise for "blaming victims." However, many established metaphysicians, such as Dr. Stuart Grayson of Manhattan's First Church of Religious Science, go to great pains in stressing that "frequently mental and physical patterns are of the unconscious or 'collective race mind,' and proceed through, but not from the patients' personal psyches" (conversation with the author 5/15/90).

In recruiting a New Age practitioner, I specifically chose a mystic who had distinguished herself through devoting many hours to volunteer work with AIDS people in hospitals and hospices. The interview was a few hours long. I extracted the most salient passages and arranged them in the following sequence with the "channeler," Nancy Karl's, express consent.

WHITEFEATHER

"We are with you," was the warm greeting. The medium is a strikingly beautiful 30-year-old of relaxed and direct demeanor. She herself is obviously an integral part of whatever wisdom she accesses through her meditations.

"It is true that AIDS, like any illness, could not be activated in the absence of some karmic pattern. But the trigger is often an imposed *judgement*. When any individual *is in agreement with* such judgement, an illness can manifest. This happens when, at that deep level where the physical and the consciousness meet, *difference* between the being and the social judgement is realized. If they [the individuals] choose to be in agreement, in any way, with any extreme judgement, then they may forfeit their immunity.''

The speaker went on to say that those with AIDS are "shocked" into releasing any agreement with negative judgements about themselves. (This may presume completed lives viewed in afterlife perspective). And with regard to contemporary moralists she imparted: *"the judgement acts as a spotlight on the judges' existences. It leads them down the path to completion where they must meet the truth of their own larger selves. This is a transformational and global aspect to the disease but all traumas have both individual and global significance."*

Enlightenings

The discussion continued to the effect that, as are the judges and the judged thus evolved, so are those in attendance and association with the PWAs: "Persons such as would never confront issues "gay" are brought into immediate contact through involvement in hospices and with friends and relatives. As the shock of an AIDS diagnosis blows apart the conditioning of the diagnosed, so the shocking fact of the disease also melts ego walls for those in attendance. In seeing PWAs as people to be 'served' rather than 'labeled', the servers can no longer be separate from 'gays'.''

Several times it was said that AIDS is the "catalyst for a transformation of consciousness." It was also said that all of these healings are permanent: *"AIDS brings to the foreground this belief in duality which judges*; The Truth wants Itself to be whole, as do all individuals. This is why we speak to you. To assist you with this. And we do speak from a place beyond duality."

I was left contemplating the bravery of such beings as might incarnate into HIV susceptibility with intent to heal the planet's dualistic pathologies. I considered the communication not unfathomable. After all, the end of philosophy is exploration, not science. Of

course, any of the various phenomena which "channelers" manifest, a change in voice, disjointed body movements, etc. (there was
none of this in the interview above), could be effected by either
theatrics or psychoses. But the electricity and integrity which ac-
company such deliveries are quite remarkable. And the *content* is
sometimes so original and inspired that I have no trouble at all acknowledging it as sourced in the spiritual realm of visions and
dreams to which so many artists and inventors freely attribute their
ideas.

Homophobia Is Bad for the Immune System

As to the particular content above, many people with HIV disease *are* from groups badly devalued by the dominant society. And
even many health professionals now acknowledge the medical importance of self love, and positive attitudes. Nor would a particular
vulnerability, experienced by gay men vs. lesbians, be incomprehensible. With the societal understanding of "masculinity's" so
closely approximating "personhood," women seen as aspiring to it
may well internalize less devaluation than men seen as renouncing
it. "Tom boys" are, in fact, often less demeaned than are "sissies." And the presumed status of physical masculinity might indeed inspire more self-censure through a "failure to live up to it"
than would the renunciation (by such women autonomous enough
to have acknowledged lesbianism), of an already badly devalued
terrain.

More was said, about the evolution of souls through contact with
their higher selves. Whitefeather said the exoteric revolution that
results from this movement can be unified by "looking within."
She repeated that the healing which comes from looking within and
meeting the higher self is "a permanent transformation" for individuals and the larger globe. Whitefeather withdrew.

A PLANETARY HISTORY OF "TRANSMISSIONS"

Weird, yes, but the Bible's full of that stuff. They heard voices
and they talked in "tongues" and many of them were certifiable by
any contemporary standards. If revelations of the past are no more

documentable than are those of the present, then neither are they more suitable for legislative implementation. The fact is that no one's psychic phenomena ought to be legislated in the United States of America. But everyone should be free to explore whatever spiritual path presents itself. And this is not possible for spiritual gays when some religions are implementing through government the idea that gender roles are absolute. Nor is it possible for spiritual humanitarians when some religions are legislating mandatory, indiscriminate reproduction.

Since moral perspectives are yet being formed respective to the revelations of two and three thousand years ago, it is necessary that such material be compared to similar present works. Because some of what's appearing today makes a hell of a lot more sense than the stuff from a time when slavery was a norm, when "sins" like menstruation commanded the sacrifice of turtledoves (Leviticus 15), and when men had to impregnate their widowed sisters-in-law.

MORE THINGS IN HEAVEN AND EARTH

Who's sure about these things anyway? Sometimes the supernatural becomes objective simply through the purview of expanding science. Psychics and artists saw the volatile human aura or 'halo" millennia before Kirlian photography, a 20th century Russian technique, confirmed the existence of just such an energy field. So science, carefully, of course, expands to admit such evidence as new technologies provide. But it can only do so if it is free enough of dogma to admit such evidence as is provable on its own terms. Auras, reincarnations, and UFOs may all revise science someday, much as did the round world and heliocentricity. But one should remember that if the orthodox church had had its way, we would still be geocentric, with dissenters executed for the pains.

Anomalous phenomena are the keys to greater knowledge. They herald the frontier, and point where to look for the future. Ships, inexplicably disappearing bottom first over the horizon, eventually told sailors the earth was round. And a 10% lesbian/gay-male incidence in the population should be telling us that "gender" is by no means the absolute it is presumed to be.

Gay persons constitute an anomaly such as casts doubt upon the presumed natural/divine basis for assigned gender roles. The proponents of mandated genderism become then as flat earthers, arguing that explorers will plunge off the edge of the world should they pursue their deviant courses. It is interesting that gay religious groups sometimes inspire the very worst in homophobic reactions among literalists. As far as they can see, the earth is flat. But they can't see very far.

NEW WINE IN OLD WINESKINS?

Will the new metaphysics relax the rubric? Perhaps, but should these mediums or their messages be either worshipped or dogmatized, then yet another *religion* will ensue, with its own orthodoxy and perhaps its own theocracy. For, alas, whatever the message, charismatic or disincarnate, it is colored by its medium. And some "channels" would cheerfully "document" to new revelations every prejudice to which the Judeo/Christian rubric has fallen heir, including an elevation of such phenomena as "creationism" and heterosexist gender roles to spiritual absolutes.

Whatever "spirit" may be, it manifests through *personalities* who interpret it according to their own belief systems and package it in conduits of their own structure. Even presupposing a "spirit" as eternal and infinite, each funnel through which it passes constrains it to that shape.

Fundamentalist funnels effect a euphoria for people whose conflicts are resolved by a belief system precluding questions and decisions. Such persons are freed from the painful necessity to think. But the enormous price they pay for their self righteousness is apparent in the mental illness which erupts among their numbers. Fundamentalists Anonymous is one recovery group designed explicitly for persons in whom fundamentalism has induced suicidal depression, bankruptcy, divorce, and violence.

F.A.

Dr. Richard Childs, a Kansas City psychiatrist who helped organize an F.A. chapter, explains: "I was thrilled to hear of Fundamentalists Anonymous, because I had been seeing patients for years suffering from their experiences with extremist religions. People had been afraid to speak up. It was like attacking the flag or Jesus himself to talk of mental problems caused by religion" (*New York Times* 4/4/87). Or as was remarked by Reverend Cristine Grimbol, a Presbyterian minister who was in early years a "charismatic" Christian: "what I didn't realize then was that the whole charismatic movement was like alcohol, an addiction that took away the pain" (*New York Times* "Long Island Interview" 11/19/89).

Pure mysticism presumes that all souls have conduits to spirit. What's in question is the shape of their funnels. What happens in dogmatism is that zealots deny the spiritual integrity of anyone whose funnel is differently shaped.

NOTHING NEW UNDER THE SUN

For example, a belief that "thoughts" translate into "things" is pro forma in much religious tradition. A pure strain of this idea is represented in Religious Science's teaching that mental events, regardless of the mental agent's denomination, are eventually represented in physical form. Jesus, likewise, taught that beliefs manifested physical events: "your faith has made you well" (Luke 8:48). And an established scientific tenet of relativity, which considers energy and matter interchangeable, perhaps gives some credence to the generalities underlying these beliefs. But literal denominations often insist that healings and demonstrations come about only if the believers observe the sect's religious requirements, i.e., not drinking, not dancing, not "being gay," etc. Instead of exploring or practicing the spirit in the funnel, they involve themselves, sometimes obsessively, with invalidating other people's funnels. Orthodox Christians light candles and say prayers expecting answers and results. But when Witches (neo-Pagans) with traditions far older than Judeo/Christianity's write "spells" on the candles and make them rhyme, the orthodoxy responds with everything from denunciation to extermination. And when polytheists see the Spirit in her many male and female guises, dogmatic Christians detect "satanism." But Catholics have at least as many saints as the Goddess has guises, some of them actually cast in plastic for the dashboard.

THE SACRED TREE

The Tree of Life was a sacred symbol millennia before anyone was nailed onto it [Churchward 88; also see illustration in photo section]. Often drawn as a "T" or "Tau" laden with foliage and avians, this cross declared the resurrection of spring. If Christ is the life force in the old Pagan tree, then all may partake. If Christ is the mistranslation of a sexist desert ritual, then Christianity is the sole province of biologic dogmatists. But such literalism may someday lose its ground. For soldiers of the literalist cross have so denied spirit to the atypical among them that the lesbian/gay-male spiritual consciousness began to grow on its own, directly, gnostically, without the church.

CHAPTER 8

ACTION!

In a final twist, gays, robbed of their god, their life force, and their freedom of speech, became one of the few groups in United States history ever specifically denied the right to association. In the absence of churches, school socialization structures, and those normal cultural patterns most U.S. residents enjoy, bars became gays' only mecca. Consequently, it became illegal in such central states as New York to serve liquor to "known homosexuals." Eventually civil disobedience dislodged this specific outrage; and gay bars emerged as churches, temples, homes, schools, and political headquarters for lesbians and gay men alike. (There is frequent conjecture that this ghettoization of gays in bars, still prevalent in many parts of the country, encourages alcohol abuse. It should be noted, however, that *alcoholism* is not a social phenomenon but rather a metabolic disease whose progression is facilitated by alcohol use.)

One of the best and best known gay bars was "Three" on New York's upper East Side, with the droll, intensely literary Anne Butler and sparkling, show-biz Jackie Scott as resident proprietor-shamans. The repartee was quicksilver and very famous people were there, some gay, some just there for the wit. Elsewhere uptown reigned Pat, Patsy, and Gwen, each presiding over a salon culture of the '50s and '60s.

Downtown, the gay bars were "raided" religiously. Such events were controlled through arrangements between police on the take and such syndicated conglomerates as tend to own "marginal" establishments. So only a few of the most atypical patrons would experience arrest and the publicity which would occasion loss of employment and housing. But always at issue was the right to association and the right to assemble, afforded through the Constitution's First Amendment. And it was the flagrant violation of this interest which directly impelled contemporary gay civil rights in the United States.

STONEWALL

The Stonewall Inn, a bar in Manhattan's Greenwich Village, hosted the inception of today's lesbian/gay-male movement. At this site, in June of 1969, the community fought back and for three days contested the intrusive, institutionalized harassment which characterizes existence for 10% of the country's population.

Two decades into the present movement, celebrations of "Stonewall 20" took place in over 80 U.S. cities. And through the efforts of the Gay & Lesbian Alliance Against Defamation, a New York-based watchdog organization, a stamp cancellation was authorized by the United States Post Office in honor of the Stonewall Rebellion.

CONSCIOUSNESS RAISING

GLAAD is an excellent example of what can be done to address the issues raised in *God's Country*. This enormously effective organization mobilizes nationwide response to anti-gay media bias through letter writing campaigns and a "PhoneTree." The efforts are particularly important in the current context of computerized right wing mailing blitzes, which attack any representation of gay men and lesbians as "healthy" or "normal" people, and which *demand* that news coverage presume an unobjective anti-gay bias. GLAAD is also credited with Bob Hope's apologizing for an anti-gay joke with a public service television spot decrying anti-gay violence.

What can also be done is for affected persons to emerge at whatever level of visibility is possible. It is important that professionals in all fields discuss current research and perspectives on these issues whose terms are now so often defined by the fringe right. Organizations can donate relevant books to libraries and affiliates. And, perhaps most importantly, individuals may counter the incessant anti-gay print media bias through letters to local editors.

EXAMPLES

Dear Editor,

Your remarks about lesbian and gay people in the June 21 Gazette editorial column were inflammatory and misleading. The traits which eventually emerge as sexual orientation are established before school age and are in no way influenced by the orientations of parents or teachers.

Ten percent of the readership's children *are* lesbian or gay. Homophobic media rhetoric increases their already staggering risk for bias violence, verbal abuse, suicide, and general discrimination.

We invite the entire community, and especially the media, to the July 4th Forum on Bias Issues which is co-sponsored by 11 local organizations and slated for 7 PM at Springdale's Main Street Community Center.

Thank you,
Springdale resident (name)

Dear Editor,

The predominance your publication affords conservative religious groups should be balanced with a dialogue about personal privacy rights. While some extremely vocal denominations wish to legislate upon others their beliefs about birth control, abortion, sexual orientation, and in vitro fertilization, these areas reflect the most intimate and profoundly private aspects of personal life.

Our country's Constitutionally mandated separation of church and state assures that all religious groups may espouse and practice their various beliefs and customs. But this same mechanism precludes the imposition of particular sectarian dogmas upon persons who either eschew religion or are members of other denominations.

Most mainstream religious groups respect church/state separation and individual privacy rights for all. We would ask that the Sun's coverage reflect this diversity.

Thank you,
Name (and any relevant affiliation)

Editor,

I protest the July 7 letter to the Editor's characterization of gays in the Pride Day parade as "flaunting homosexuality." Non-gays flaunt their sexualities religiously, in a ritualized norm which is so widespread as to have become invisible. Marriages, wedding rings, "Mr. & Mrs." designations, and airport goodbye kisses are ubiquitous brandishings of orientation. Heterosexist insistence upon suppression of these expressions among lesbians and gays is a profound violation of Constitutional rights. Free speech is entirely precluded when discrimination based on one's private life necessitates deception.

Thank you,
Name

Note: Please, with express permission of the author, feel free to adapt or reproduce the above letters for local use. The letter writer's name, address, and telephone number should always be included so that the publishers may verify authorship. One may note that address and phone are not for publication.

ORGANIZATION

Today a vast network of educational and cultural recourse is available to the gay community. Special organizations serve lesbian and gay Asians, Latins, Catholics, and Native Americans. The National Coalition for Black Lesbians and Gays (Washington, DC) has been in service since 1978. Another resource is the American Civil Liberties Union (ACLU) whose state and local affiliates (NYCLU and NYCLU-Suffolk) were all-important in the Suffolk county civil rights effort. Generally, educational efforts activate allies who had previously not understood the depth of the problem, simply because, as heterosexuals, they had never been targets of homophobia. As for structure in the larger civil liberties arena, many national organizations have active regional affiliates and the National Abortion Rights Action League (NARAL of Washington, DC) publishes a Reproductive Rights Issues Manual to guide local efforts.

The contemporary emphasis on lesbian and gay male visibility was greatly consolidated at 1988's Washington, DC conference of gay community leaders. One outgrowth was the widespread media presence of National Coming Out Day. Now an independent enterprise, this event was originally spearheaded by the California-based public interest law firm National Gay Rights Advocates. Another group, SAGE, operating out of Manhattan's Lesbian & Gay Community Services Center, is an educational and service organization specifically for lesbian/gay seniors. The Lesbian Herstory Archives in New York City is a fast growing institution. And many regions now have chapters of the Washington-based Federation of Parents and Friends of Lesbians and Gays. This group has proved an invaluable resource, and Long Island P-FLAG was a beacon of community awareness during the Suffolk County rights bill hearings.

LINGUISTIC STRATEGIES

The single most powerful consciousness-raising tool is, perhaps, the language which conducts our thoughts. And great linguistic strides, some already discussed, have been taken by the gay/feminist movements. It is useful to become aware of the ways in which word habits foster and perpetuate negative stereotypes. Linguistic strategies have been devised to reverse those trends. For example, the change from "maiden name" to "birth name" helps eradicate the idea of a pedestalized virginity presumed exclusively for women. And feminist Gloria Steinem's rescue of the secretarial caption "Ms." from 19th century obscurity redresses the injustice of marital status as an exclusive designation for women.

"Lady" is now juxtaposed with "gentleman" but not "man" to defeat the pedestalizing "men and ladies." "Girl" is declined for adult women, in so far as it suggests, condescendingly, that the aging process which is so distinguishing and prestigious in men, is a negative among females.

Also, a particularly dramatic symbol has been reclaimed in recent decades for political and educational purposes. The Nazi regime incarcerated and executed many thousands of gays under the auspices of The Federal Security Office for Combating Abortion and Homosexuality, established in 1936 [Plant 86]. The pink triangle insigne gay people were forced to wear in the concentration camps has become a crest at many contemporary lesbian and gay events. And the epithetical "dyke" has been proudly repossessed by many lesbians.

Some linguistic activists refuse to use the term "couple" in reference to straights without the adjective "heterosexual," in that the term has been so commandeered as the exclusive province of non-gays. Others decline participation in the "weddings" which confer upon heterosexual unions a privileged status denied lesbians and gay men.

Also significant is that the language, being a construct of the patriarchy, is not rich in ungendered terms. The generic "he," "man," and "mankind" have long been obsolete in "politically correct" circles, with "the human race" and "humanity" replacing some such terms. But gays are often still adrift for designations as members of couples.

Solve This Problem!

Unsolved problems are represented by terms like "spouse," which presumes a legal status gays do not yet enjoy. The very common "lover" sometimes implies an impermanence or predominant physicality which is not appropriate. "Partner" sounds financial, and "mate" conjures up images zoological. The author sometimes uses "complement" which perhaps implies a degree of "better half" interdependence touching on psychological ill health.

The absence of a gender-neutral personal pronoun makes the language itself hierarchal because in a patriarchy, gendered terms are themselves hierarchal. Suggestions arise, from time to time, as to how to remedy this linguistic deficit. Perhaps the New Age would countenance "en" (to replace he or she), in honor of the interdimensional "entity" presumed transcendent of gendered incarnations. "Entity" is, after all, defined as "the essence of something apart from its accidental properties." The possessive would reduce "her" and "his" to "es" (pronounced "s") with the objective also "en," giving rise to the form "enself."

BROAD IMPLICATIONS

It would be almost impossible to exaggerate the extent to which a release from the reflexive grip of sexist thought could heal what is wrong within the U.S. and elsewhere. Mindless pronatalism steers the world to a population catastrophe while women attempting to control their fertility are thwarted, maimed, and killed. Finite taxpayer resources are absorbed to artificially sustain bodies in irreversible vegetative conditions. Meanwhile, the hungry stay hungry. Over and over it has been shown that a patriarchy subjugating half its own race does not hesitate to imprison the whole of another. And the planetary stage upon which these tragedies unfold is expanding wildly in toxicity, even as the ascendance of technological progress excludes just such intuitive connections with nature as might preserve her works.

In this demise does the United States of America lead the fray, particularly as to sexist specifics. At home, the phobias which exacerbate AIDS continue to stifle education and in doing so kill, literally, thousands of people. The same sentiments make suicide the likeliest of deaths among the 10% of the country's youth. The numbers of homeless and abused children is a momentous disgrace. Yet the U.S. government remains formally committed to mandated childbirth both here and abroad.

REVOKE THEIR DIPLOMATIC IMMUNITY!

Homophobic and gynephobic institutions are dangerous and should be identified thus in exactly the same ways as are neo-Nazis and the Ku Klux Klan. The latter organizations in no way enjoy the polite editorial immunity often afforded Catholics and fundamentalists.

For example, when on December 11, 1989, women's and AIDS groups protested in Manhattan's St. Patrick's Cathedral, the media was lavish in coverage of official "outrage" about disturbing a religious service. But the Catholic Church has consistently disturbed the spiritual, psychological, and physical well-being of women for two thousand years. No mention was made of the outrage that Cardinal O'Connor had voiced support for Operation Rescue, the terrorist group which, nationwide, barricades sites providing to women the spiritual sine qua non of reproductive autonomy. And the Cardinal certainly does not confine his influence to religious spheres. He has actually served on a governmental commission for the formulation of AIDS policy. Explaining that his sworn allegiance to the Vatican precludes independent judgment, this man's official input is to *oppose* safer sex wherewithall and information in adamance that only those kinds of sex his church approves should be non-fatal throughout the world.

TAX-EXEMPT BEHEMOTHS

That luminary tax-exempt goliaths are permitted to effect removal of protections from the country's most violated groups is a national disgrace. Although free speech presumes every group's right to expression, religious status should not authorize bigots to form national policies. Religious status did not excuse the crusades and witch burnings of the past, and it should not excuse the genocides of today.

Patriarchy has commandeered universals and instructed women and gays to access those universals through heterosexual men. If the New Age is new at all it will facilitate universals as immediately accessible to all beings. And the same key unlocks the outside and the inside of the door, for from spiritual autonomy springs wisdom, invention, strategy, communication, and effectiveness.

The religious right's arguments about civil liberties' destroying the country have been used against every significant rights increment from women's suffrage to the integrated army. Women have a right to any autonomy claimed by men. And to extreme planetary detriment does the male dominated culture eschew the intuitive faculty it delegates to women. These are truths.

True also is the fact that heterosexuality is neither a norm nor an objective value, and the militant insistence upon its acquisition is destructive to a great many people.

EPILOGUE

It is, perhaps, relevant to this conclusion that the *God's Country* character vignettes which employ first and last names do so with the subjects' express permission. An exception is Brad's sketch, which is anonymous for the somber reason that the man interviewed did not survive to approve the final draft. Although he had not requested anonymity, he did ask to see the passage and out of respect his surname is withheld. What is particularly disturbing is that the specific HIV-related complication to which Brad succumbed is now being kept at bay for increasingly longer periods of time. It is very conceivable that, absent the homophobic shroud obscuring AIDS, today's advances might have become available in such time as to have considerably extended Brad's active life.

This irrationality surrounding the AIDS pandemic is just one more indication that the gender polarization experiment of the last three millennium has failed. If the land of the free and the brave intends to figure at all in the resolution of this failure, she had best engage reason, rather than doctrine, in the formulation of her national policies.

BIBLIOGRAPHY

Ballou 85 Mary Ballou, PhD and Nancy W. Gabalac, MEd. *A Feminist Position on Mental Health*. Charles C Thomas Publisher: Springfield, IL ©1985 p 102.

Bell 78 Alan P. Bell, PhD and Martin S. Weinberg, PhD. *Homosexualities*. Simon and Schuster: New York ©1978 p 60.

Bell 81 Alan P. Bell, Martin S. Weinberg, Sue Kiefer Hammersmith. *Sexual Preference*. Alfred C. Kinsey Institute for Sex Research, Indiana University Press: Bloomington, ©1981.

Benjamin 84 Jessica Benjamin, PhD. "The Convergence of Psychoanalysis and Feminism" *Women Therapists Working With Women*, Editor Claire M. Brody, PhD. Springer Publishing Company: New York ©1984.

Berlitz 84 Charles Berlitz. *Atlantis*. Putnam's: New York ©1984.

Berzon 88 Betty Berzon, PhD. *Permanent Partners*. E. P. Dutton: New York ©1988 p 47.

Bible *Holy Bible: Revised Standard Version*. Nelson and Sons: New York 1952.

Boswell 80 John Boswell. *Christianity, Social Tolerance, and Homosexuality*. University of Chicago Press: Chicago ©1980 p 92.

Brody 85 Leslie Brody, PhD. "Gender Differences in Emotional Development" *Gender and Personality*, Editors Abigail J. Stewart and M. Brinton Lykes. Duke University Press: Durham 1985.

Calderone 77 Mary S. Calderone, MD. "Of Dade County, Homosexuals, and Rights" *SIECUS Report* Vol. VI No. 1 Sept 1977.

Camp 87 Sharon Camp, PhD. "The Impact of the Mexico City Policy on Women and Health Care in Developing Countries" *Journal of International Law and Politics*. New York University; Vol. 20:35 #1 Fall 1987 p 47.

Campbell 59 Joseph Campbell. *The Masks of God: Primitive Mythology*. Viking Press: New York 1959 p 387.

Chesler 72 Phyllis Chesler, PhD. *Women and Madness*. Doubleday and Company: Garden City, New York 1972.

Churchward 88 Colonel James Churchward. *The Lost Continent of Mu*. BE Books/Brotherhood of Life: Albuquerque, NM 1988 p 146-47.

Daly 78 Mary Daly (holds doctorates in theology and philosophy from the University of Fribourg, Switzerland). *Gyn/Ecology*. Beacon Press: Boston ©1978 p 134-152.

Durant 42 Will Durant. *The Story of Civilization*. Simon and Schuster: New York Vol 1 1942 p 30-35.

Falwell 76 Reverend Jerry Falwell: Special Service 7/4/76; see Dr. William R. Goodman Jr. and Dr. James J. H. Price. *Jerry Falwell: An Unauthorized Profile*. Paris and Associates Inc: Lynchburg VA © 1981 p 91; see also [People For 82 p 54].

Falwell 81 Reverend Jerry Falwell: Fundraising letter 8/13/81, quoted in [People For 82 p 239]; for letter reprint see [Young 82 p 307].

Frankfort 79 Ellen Frankfort and Frances Kissling. *Rosie: The Investigation of a Wrongful Death*. Dial Press: New York ©1979.

Freud 05 "Three Essays on the Theory of Sexuality" *Standard Edition of the Complete Psychological Works of Sigmund Freud*, Editor James Strachey. Hogarth Press: London ©1953-1974: 7:123-246.

Freud 20 "The Psychogenesis of a Case of Homosexuality in a Woman" *Standard Edition of the Complete Psychological Works of Sigmund Freud*, Editor James Strachey. Hogarth Press: London ©1953-1974; 18:155-172.

Freud 21 Sigmund Freud; Letter (to Jones) *Body Politic*. Toronto, Canada; May 1977 p 9.

Friedan 63 Betty Friedan. *The Feminine Mystique*. W. W. Norton and Company Inc. New York 1963 p 103-125.

Grahn 84 Judy Grahn. *Another Mother Tongue*. Beacon Press: Boston 1984 p 275.

Green 87 Richard Green, MD, JD. *The "Sissy Boy Syndrome" and the Development of Homosexuality*. Yale University Press: New Haven and London 1987.

Greenberg 86 David F. Greenberg, professor of sociology at New

York University: *People* interview on Hardwick decision 7/21/86 Vol 26, No. 3 p 87.

Guttmacher 88 *Family Planning Perspectives*. Alan Guttmacher Institute: New York.

   3/88 Vol 20 No. 2 Mar/Apr 1988 p 55.

   7/88 Vol 20 No. 4 July/Aug 1988 p 168.

Harrison 85 Beverly Wildung Harrison, PhD. *Making the Connections*, Editor Carol S. Robb. Beacon Press: Boston ©1985 p 15.

Heiman 75 Julia R. Heiman, PhD. "Women's Sexual Arousal" *Psychology Today*. April 1975.

Hetrick 88 Emery S. Hetrick, MD and A. Damien Martin, EdD, New York University "The Stigmatization of the Gay and Lesbian Adolescent" in *The Treatment of Homosexuals With Mental Health Disorders*, Editor Michael W. Ross, PhD. Harrington Park Press Inc: New York ©1988.

Hooker 57 Evelyn Hooker, PhD. "The Adjustment of the Male Overt Homosexual" *Journal of Projective Techniques* 21:18-31 1957.

Hunter 84 Joyce Hunter, MSW and A. Damien Martin, EdD "A Comparison of the Presenting Problems of Homosexually and Non-homosexually Oriented Young People." ©1984 unpublished.

Hurst 83 Jane Hurst, PhD. *History of Abortion in the Catholic Church*. Catholics For a Free Choice: Washington DC 1983 p 12-20.

Interpreter's Dictionary of the Bible Abingdon Press: New York ©1962.

Kinsey 48 Alfred C. Kinsey, Wardell B. Pomeroy, Clyde E. Martin. "Homosexual Outlet" in *Sexual Behavior in the Human Male*. W. B. Saunders Company: Philadelphia ©1948.

Kinsey 53 Institute for Sex Research staff, Indiana University (Alfred C. Kinsey, Wardell B. Pomeroy, Clyde E. Martin, Paul H. Gebhard). "Homosexual Responses and Contacts" and "Anatomy of Sexual Response and Orgasm" in *Sexual Behavior in the Human Female*. W. B. Saunders Company: Philadelphia 1953.

Klaich 74 Dolores Klaich. *Woman Plus Woman*. Simon and Schuster Inc: New York 1974; The Naiad Press: Tallahasse 1989.

Lems 80 Kristin Lems. "How Nice" — "In the Out Door" album.

Carolsdatter Productions: 221-C Dodge Ave., Evanston, IL 1980.

Lewes 88 Kenneth Lewes, PhD. *The Psychoanalytic Theory of Male Homosexuality*. Simon and Schuster: New York 1988.

Marmor 65 Judd Marmor, MD. "Introduction" to *Sexual Inversion: The Multiple Roots of Homosexuality*. Basic Books Inc: New York ©1965.

Marmor 80 Judd Marmor, MD (Editor). *Homosexual Behavior: A Modern Reappraisal* Basic Books Inc: New York ©1980 p 19-20.

Martin 82 A. Damien Martin, EdD. "Learning to Hide: The Socialization of the Gay Adolescent" *Adolescent Psychiatry: Developmental and Clinical Studies* Vol X (Editors Sherman C. Feinstein, John G. Looney, Allan Z. Schwartzberg and Arthur D. Sorosky). University of Chicago 1982.

Mohr 78 James C. Mohr (Professor of History, University of Maryland). *Abortion in America*. Oxford University Press: New York 1978 p 160-170.

Money 76 John Money, PhD. "Statement on Antidiscrimination Regarding Sexual Orientation" *SIECUS Report* Sept 1977.

Money 80 John Money, PhD. *Love and Love Sickness*. Johns Hopkins University Press: Baltimore ©1980 p 33.

Money 85 John Money, PhD. *The Destroying Angel*. Prometheus Books: Buffalo, New York 1985.

Money 88 John Money, PhD. *Gay, Straight and In-Between*. Oxford University Press: New York 1988 p 49.

Morris 74 Jan Morris. *Conundrum*. Harcourt Brace Jovanovich Inc: New York 1974 p 189.

Morokoff 88 Patricia J. Morokoff, PhD: presentation at American Psychological Association meeting Atlanta, GA and *New York Times* 8/23/88.

Moses 86 A. Elfin Moses, DSW and Robert O. Hawkins Jr., PhD. *Counseling Lesbian Women and Gay Men*. Merrill Publishing Company: Columbus, OH ©1986 pp 42 & 52.

Near 79 Holly Near. "Singing For Our Lives" Hereford Music "Lifeline" album; Redwood Records: Oakland CA ©1979.

New Catholic Encyclopedia The Catholic University of America: Washington, DC ©1967.

Orwell 49 George Orwell. *1984*. Harcourt, Brace and Company: New York ©1949 p 17.

Pagels 79 Elaine Pagels, PhD. *The Gnostic Gospels*. Random House: New York ©1979 p 124.

Pattison 80 E. Mansell Pattison, MD and Myrna Loy Pattison. "'Ex-Gays': Religiously Mediated Change in Homosexuals" *American Journal of Psychiatry* 137:12; December 1980.

People For 82 People For The American Way: Washington DC; David Bollier *Liberty and Justice For Some*. Frederick Ungar Publishing Company: New York ©1982.

People For 88 *Attacks on the Freedom to Learn: The 1987-1988 Report*. People For The American Way: Washington DC; see also *New York Times* 9/1/88.

Plant 86 Richard Plant. *The Pink Triangle*. Henry Holt and Company: New York 1986 p 149.

Rapp 89 Sandy Rapp. "Remember Rose: A Song For Choice" Sandy Rapp Music: Sag Harbor, New York 1989.

RCAR Religious Coalition for Abortion Rights: Washington DC.
   87 "Religious Freedom and the Abortion Controversy" 5/87.
   88 "Options" Spring 1988 p 4.
   90 "We Affirm" 3/90.

Roberts 79 Jane Roberts. *The Nature Of The Psyche*. Bantam: New York ©1979 p 76-90.

Robertson 81 Reverend Pat Robertson: "700 Club" broadcast 12/20/81; quoted in [People For 82 p 258].

Robinson 77 James M. Robinson (Editor). *The Nag Hammadi Library*. Harper and Row: San Francisco ©1977 (Revised Edition ©1988).

Rodegast 85 Pat Rodegast and Judith Stanton. *Emmanuel's Book*. Bantam: New York ©1985 p 227.

Schlafly 81 Phyllis Schlafly quoted in the Philadelphia *Daily News* 7/2/81; see also [People For 82 p 238].

Silverstein 77 Charles Silverstein, PhD. *A Family Matter*. Mc-Graw-Hill Book Company: New York ©1977.

Sitchin 78 Zecharia Sitchin. *The 12th Planet*. Avon: New York ©1978 p 105.

Socarides 70 Charles W. Socarides, MD. "Homosexuality and

Medicine" *JAMA: The Journal of the American Medical Association* May 18, 1970 Vol. 212 No 7.

Stephenson 81 June Stephenson, PhD. *Women's Roots*. Diemer, Smith Pub: Napa, CA ©1981 p 15-22.

Stone 76 Merlin Stone. *When God Was a Woman*. Harcourt Brace Jovanovich Inc.: New York ©1976 p 158-9 & 195.

Terry 88 Randall Terry. *Philadelphia Inquirier* interview 6/26/88; quoted by Planned Parenthood Federation of America in "Time" magazine advertisement 2/6/89 p 37.

Von Rad 61 Gerhard Von Rad. *Genesis: A Commentary* translation by John Marks. Westminster Press: Philadelphia ©1961 p 120.

Wink 79 Dr. Walter Wink: presentation at New York Annual Conference meeting, Memorial United Methodist Church, White Plains, New York 1/23/79.

Wright 82 Ezekiel Wright and Daniel Inesse. *God Is Gay*. Tayu Press: Santa Rosa CA ©1982 p 86 & 87.

Young 82 Perry Deane Young. *God's Bullies*. Holt, Rinehart and Winston: New York ©1982 p 307 (8/13/81 Falwell mailing reprint).

ZPG 90 "An Uncompromising Position" *ZPG Backgrounder* Zero Population Growth: Washington DC June 1990.

Zwerin 87 Rabbis Raymond A. Zwerin and Richard J. Shapiro. *Judaism and Abortion*. Religious Coalition for Abortion Rights: Washington DC 1987.

Index

ABOUT THE AUTHOR

Sandy Rapp is a grassroots gay/lesbian and women's rights activist. She has been instrumental in the development and passage of several gay civil rights measures and, under the auspices of Long Island's East End Gay Organization, has conducted gay/lesbian sensitivity training for the Suffolk County Police Department and co-chaired an extensive series of forums on AIDS and civil liberties. Ms. Rapp, a musician by trade, currently gives rights talks and feminist guitar/vocal concerts. She received an MA from the University of Aberdeen in Scotland.